Hemip

afte.

or

Traumatic Brain Injury

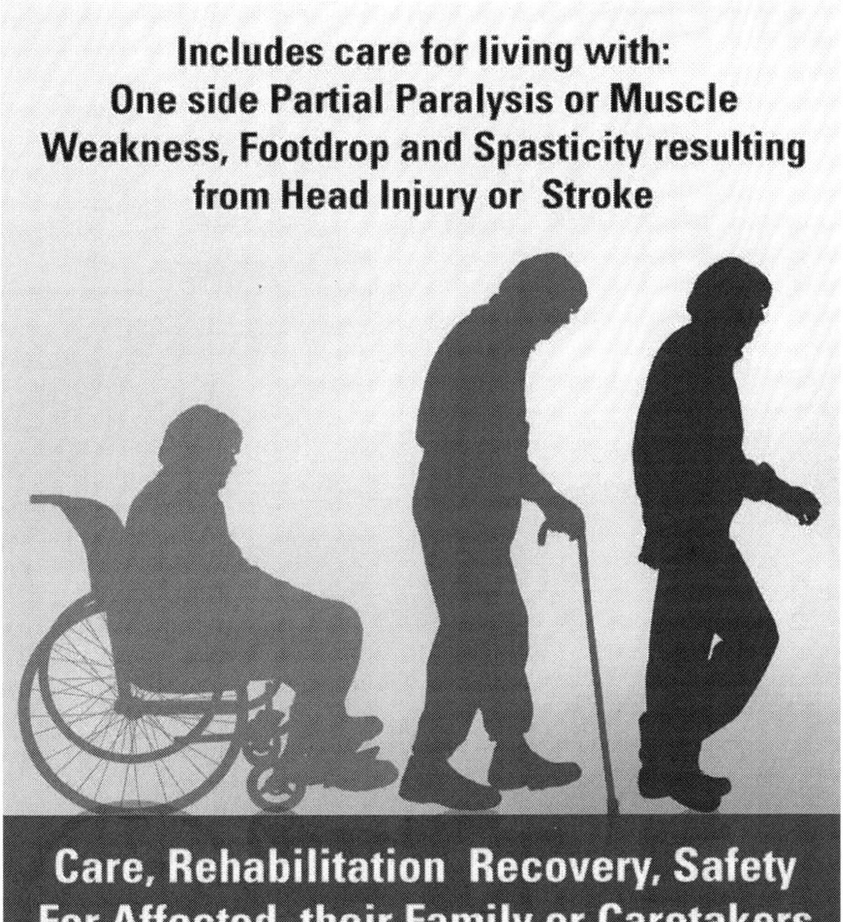
Includes care for living with:
One side Partial Paralysis or Muscle
Weakness, Footdrop and Spasticity resulting
from Head Injury or Stroke
Care, Rehabilitation Recovery, Safety
For Affected, their Family or Caretakers

Leon Edward

DEDICATION

Helping families and loved ones understand care after a brain injury or stroke with hemiparesis and assisting the injured in rehabilitation and safety is a passion of the author, Leon Edward who has spent over three decades successfully living with effects as hemiparesis after traumatic brain injury being shot in the head and neck.

"This is written with a deep care for my brothers and sisters affected as I have been, plus their families and/or caretakers."

Contents

ACKNOWLEDGMENTS

I am so greatly thankful for the expert treatment and care from the physicians, nurses, physical therapists, occupational therapists, the vocational therapists that worked with me on my re-entry into living, working, social environments.

I am thankful for the peace from God above and the help guiding me to provide this resource and subsequent series that would be helpful not only for affected loved ones but most importantly for the safety and living of the injured.

Introduction

Our lives can change drastically in moments when there is either a stroke or traumatic brain injury leaving yourself or a loved one with hemiparesis, where a side of your body is partially paralyzed or exhibits extreme muscle weakness. Other issues associated with this type of injury or condition as foot drop and spasticity are also reviewed in this book for care, rehabilitation, safety and generally living successfully.

Hemiparesis can be the result of many types of conditions and injuries. Hemiparesis can be caused in several ways as detailed in the first chapter. As an introduction, most causes of hemiparesis are due to injury to the brain, from loss of oxygen. While the main cause of hemiparesis is due to a stroke, in which there is a loss of blood to a part of the brain. Other causes of hemiparesis include: trauma/falls, tumors, traumatic brain injuries, congenital defects, or birth injuries.

The time spent in hospitals or care centers may be shorter these days with one's specific health plan coverage as is more common than not. Home care exercise and follow-up improvement is going to be very important as rehabilitation continues as you succeed in your recovery.

Also, is important to note briefly here that recovery varies significantly amongst individuals but the information and tips provided in this book are intended and proven to instill practices, habits, some exercises of body and mind to succeed in your life no matter what limitations you may have and live even better than what others consider a normal life.

That being stated, by reviewing the contents section, the approach to this guide is to clearly and succinctly describe the possible effects, known rehabilitation and care at home with an emphasis on safety concerns. This guide can also give your insight on what can be expected living with hemiparesis, muscle weakness or partial paralysis, foot drop, spasticity or as myself over the years, all effects listed to a degree.

Besides the must have basic care and rehabilitation information, real value of this book is the passing on of real life experiences and insights. As a person successfully living, working for over 30 years with hemiparesis, I also can offer personal insights of my own experiences and yes, some lessons learned too. Although, some of my comments may seem mundanely simple or obvious, many are safety tips that may prevent serious accidental injury. Some stories of experience may even seem funny especially if from an experience familiar to you or from a loved one.

It is important to note that the best care, advice, recommendations, re-training of mind and body is from your health professionals and even more so specifically for each person's individual or unique case.

Let me be clear in this introduction that I am an engineer not a medical doctor nor other health professional but where I've researched the field and I can, add references to assist others in their recovery, I have with an added resource section. I feel this reference and resource section is invaluable improvement since when I was first affected leaving my family unsure of what damage short term or long term exactly, what changes were there, what would happen, who to talk to… and without many references or even website forums to communicate with others affected. The current availability of organizations that can assist, personal groups in forums or even Facebook just didn't exist at that time outside of the hospitals and care centers. This guide and the authors website will provide these needed associations now with updates available ongoing on the website as referenced in the resource section

In writing this book, researching information, facts, updates in care, I realized that what be my best research was living through this for the past few decades. As I wrote this book and researched current facts, treatments with individual experiences from others affected, I realized that living through initial rehabilitation in the hospital, after being in a coma, then a lengthy rehabilitation program leading to partial recovery followed by decades living with hemiparesis effects could in effect be a blessing to help others affected and their families in primarily the safety of my affected brothers and sisters. Yes, stroke survivors, disabled or brain injured similarly can often form strong bonds from going through similar struggles and accomplishments.

In these over 30 years, conditions lessened, improved, caused a few injuries with subsequent rehabilitation several times after setbacks for one reason or another. I can even say I have become good at rehabilitation after injuries or weakening from an illness or weather conditions. Although, gyms, swimming pools and at home exercising became the norm in my schedule. I'll share my physical therapists and textbook recommendations generalized plus a few timesaving and safety recommendations from lessons learned.

Sections offer tips interspersed with some of these unique insights but also at times where it may add value, sharing some of my emotions and feelings hoping that these may be beneficial to others and their families who experience a sudden life change as when one is affected by hemiparesis, hemiplegia or extreme muscle weakness, even partial paralysis on a side of the body.

Eventually becoming a successful engineer years after my own physical and mental rehabilitation, I am competent researcher of facts and often analyzed issues throughout recovery process and about rehabilitation, care, safety.

Also, I was naturally curious about understanding everything I was experiencing with my sudden injury or weakness and through the years, I've also learned from top health professionals, while making and survived my own mistakes. My passion after graduate school became understanding cognitive difficulties and improving brain functions. I add small sections throughout the book where my research in brain science, neuroplasticity effects, audio effects on the brain may be value added in improving cognitive functioning including, concentration, focus, attention, improving memory, recall and socially interactions or behavior. Of course, one's own physician and health professionals would be needed to be referred to at least on any audio or visual stimulation.

I will add my own insights throughout the main content and some added published articles on living with hemiparesis issues and concerns in the appendix for reference. Many of the insights, my own comments, tips, techniques are intended towards the person living with hemiparesis, while the overall review of care and rehabilitation is for them and for and their family members or caretakers. Plus, myself, with an engineering and statistical problem-solving education and background have examined situations so as often be analytical in my examination and overcoming issues.

As I added sections, more and more came to mind on how I felt at certain periods of my life and people reactions. From family members to friends, to colleagues and in business, communication and interactions experience can provide others affected with insights that would be beneficial to them. Also, motivation, encouragement, self-esteem, maintaining positive attitude, successful traits, self-improvement by myself and others who have gone through this and succeeded are some ideas for future books from this author. Check out me about section near the end of this book, and sign up free for news on future releases and discounts.

- Leon Edward

Overview of Hemiparesis and Associated Conditions

Hemiparesis is a medical term that refers to weakness in one side of the body. "Hemi" means *half* and "paresis" means *weakness*. It is also associated with the medical term hemiplegia, which means paralysis of one side of the body. For individuals affected with hemiparesis, there is still movement of the affected side of the body but with less strength. One sided weakness can affect the arms, hands, legs and muscles of the face. This weakness impacts the ability to perform daily activities, self-care tasks and walking.

Other common impairments associated with hemiparesis include:

- Balance limitations
- Inability to walk or walking instability
- Limited control of hand function and grip strength
- Impaired coordination and control of precise movements
- Fatigue
- Decreased overall independence

Hemiparesis can be the result of many types of conditions and injuries. Most causes of hemiparesis are due to injury to the brain, from loss of oxygen. The main cause of hemiparesis is due to a stroke, in which there is a loss of blood to a part of the brain. Other causes of hemiparesis include: trauma/falls, tumors, traumatic brain injuries, congenital defects, or birth injuries.

The brain is the powerhouse of the central nervous system and all the bodies functions. The brain is connected to the spinal cord and peripheral nerves leave the spinal cord to innervate the rest of the body. The brain sends signals via nerves to the entire body, controlling all movement and sensations. If there is injury to one part of the brain, then it cannot properly send nerve signals and create movement. This disruption of brain function is why muscle strength is lost. There is no injury to the muscle, but the signal for activation has been lost or diminished.

The location in which the brain injury occurs will determine where the weakness will present. If there is injury to the left side of the brain (which controls speaking and language), it can result in weakness to the right side of the body and negatively affect communication. If there is injury to the right side of the brain, left sided weakness can result. For some brain injuries (though less likely), weakness will be on the same side of injury.

Throughout this book, this condition will be referred to as hemiparesis weakness of muscles on one side for consistency but similar conditions, effects are exhibited in partial paralysis, paralysis can be identified more specifically and accurately by your health professionals based on an individual's specific cause and effects.

Associated Conditions

Hemiplegia or hemiplegia/ (-ple´jah) paralysis of one side of the body.

Alternate (or crossed) paralysis of one side of the face and the opposite side of the body.

Cerebral hemiplegia that due to a brain lesion.

Facial hemiplegia paralysis of one side of the face.

Spastic hemiplegia hemiplegia with spasticity of the affected muscles and Increased tendon reflexes.

Spinal hemiplegia that due to a lesion of the spinal cord.

Stroke (Cerebral Vascular Accident)

A stroke is a sudden loss of neurologic function in the brain, caused by an interruption of blood flow to the brain. Strokes can be a result of ischemic or hemorrhagic infarcts. An ischemic stroke is one in which a clot blocks blood flow, depriving the brain of needed oxygen. Ischemic strokes are the most common type, accounting for approximately 80% of strokes. Hemorrhagic strokes happen when blood vessels rupture, leaking blood in and around the brain.

Stroke is the third leading cause of death and most common cause of disability in adults of the United States. As of this writing, it affects 700,000 individuals each year, with 500,000 new cases and 200,000 recurrent strokes. It is estimated that there are 5,400,000 stroke survivors, which accounts for 2.6 percent of the population in the United States. Men are more likely to suffer strokes than women, and African Americans, Mexican-Americans, and American Indians have a higher risk of stroke as compared to Caucasians. Stroke is the most common cause of chronic disability in the U.S. For survivors, 1/3 are functionally dependent after 1 year, meaning they need assistance with daily activities, walking, and/or speech. Approximately 26% of patients with stroke are in a nursing home institution.

After onset of stroke, there are many common clinical findings, including: changes in consciousness, impairment to the sensory and motor systems, as well as changes to the perceptual and language functions. Hemiparesis typically occurs on the side of the body that is opposite the site of brain injury. The brain functions in a manner that motor tasks and sensation crosses the medulla (middle of the brain) to control the opposite side of the body. The location and extent of brain injury, as well as acute management are huge determinants in the long-term severity of neurologic deficits.

Motor function is the most commonly affected neurologic side effect of stroke. Motor function is the body's ability to control movement. Weakness is found in 80-90% of all patients after stroke. Weakness is classified as the individual's inability to generate the force necessary for controlling or initiating movement.

Typically, after stroke, flaccid paralysis is present immediately. This is because of shock to the brain. Flaccid paralysis is the inability to elicit any movement. It is typically short-lived, lasting days or weeks. Flaccidity can persist in a small number of patients.

Spasticity comes about in about 90% of cases and happens in the side opposite the brain lesion. Spasticity is high tone in muscles. It results in tight/stiff muscles and limits voluntary movement. Whether muscle tone is flaccid or spastic, muscle weakness typically prevails. <u>Later in this book, an entire section is devoted to care, rehabilitation and issues of living with and overcoming spasticity</u> with exercises for at home.

Other Types of Brain Injury

Another way to acquire hemiparesis is with a head injury, because of trauma or fall. The mechanism of injury is the same as a stroke. With a head trauma, blood is pooled in one portion of the brain, injuring nervous tissue function. It is estimated that 1.5 to 2 million people incur a traumatic brain injury each year. Motor vehicle accidents and falls account for most injuries. Forces on the brain include acceleration, deceleration and rotational strain to the brain tissue against the bony skull. Depending on the area of damage, different areas of muscle strength will be affected. Spinal cord injuries due to trauma or tumors, can also damage neurologic structures, causing paralysis or weakness. Tumors can press on brain structures, causing hemiparesis or hemiplegia. Congenital conditions or birth accidents (like cerebral palsy) can also cause hemiparesis.

Widespread problem Areas

For individuals that are affected with weakness in the upper body, it is common to develop shoulder subluxation. Because of decreased muscle tone in the muscles of the shoulder, the homers (top bone in the arm) can begin to pull down, out of the shoulder socket. This subluxation can be painful, or it can happen without any discomfort. Upper arm slings, taping, as well as electric stimulation of the muscle can all help prevent or correct for subluxation.

For individuals affected with leg weakness, it is common to develop a "foot drop." A foot drop is a result of inability to control the anterior tibialis muscle, which lies over the front of the lower leg, next to the shin. This weakness leads to an inability to clear the foot when walking. The toe drags and causes a huge risk for falling. To compensate for this weakness, ankle foot orthoses can be worn. This brace supports the foot and ankle, providing rigidity and preventing the toe from dragging. Foot drop care, rehabilitation is addressed in much more needed detail in its own section later in this book.

Inability to fully open the hand is common for people that develop spasticity in their upper body. Because of the high muscle tone in the arm and hand, it is common to lose the ability to fully open the hand. It is essential that the patient pay attention to range of motion in the hand. If spasticity begins, the patient should always hold a small ball in their palm, to keep the hand open and prevent contracture in the palm.

Other Possible Side Effects

Besides loss of muscle strength, there are other unpleasant side effects of brain injury including:

Sensation loss: Sensation is commonly impaired on the affected side. This can create a changing sensation for light touch or sharp touch and temperature sensation. A change in sensation can lead to neglect for the affected side. Unilateral neglect is a situation in which the affected individual has little awareness of the hemiplegic side of the body, resulting in potential injury to that side. Personally, I have cut myself on my foot during a foot drop dragging incident and didn't realize it was cut until removing my shoe later in the day. Be careful here.

Pain: Pain is an unfortunate side effect for some individuals after a brain injury. Some experience constant, burning pain with stabbing, sharp pains. Sometimes light pressure or loud noises can elicit painful responses. Pain is also common at joint structures or in muscles with increased muscle tone.

Depending on the severity a neurologist may prescribe medication for management of the pain or discomfort. Myself, I've learned to deal with this with meditation practices and I've learned I start each day with a 15-minute meditation practice and the end my day with a 10-minute meditation practice. In the early years after my injury, I had limited medication prescribed for pain but back in often make a person drowsy I find as many others meditation helps.

There are also guided meditations and relaxation exercises available on audio and will be references in the appendix.

Vision changes: Visual changes can occur after a stroke, depending on what part of the brain structure is affected. One part of the field of vision can be lost, or patients can have visual neglect, difficulty with depth perception and spatial relationships.

Cognitive impairments: If the cognitive processing area of the brain has been injured, it can cause changes in memory and cognition. Memory problems are often very disruptive for people with brain injury. It can be very frustrating for us not being able to recall quickly. I know it can be embarrassing and causes some very awkward moments. If the injured can use humor better, it puts most everyone at ease.

More tips and training, improvement offered later in this book in care and tips sections. The importance of concentration and focus in improving cognitive processes and physical movement really requires its own section and a chapter will be devoted to this topic with exercises later in the book.

Speech impairments: Aphasia is a medical term that refers to a disruption in speech or the ability to understand verbal communication. Some individuals have difficulty speaking and difficulty expressing themselves verbally. In other individuals, there is difficulty understanding what others are trying to say. After excellent work with a speech therapists in a hospital; clarity of speech improved immensely. I must note that there should be verbal communication exercised ongoing as not all of us are conversationalists or have families around daily to practice in common communication. As an engineer living alone for years when my daughter was not around, much time was spent not communicating verbally. Even coworkers, relatives and friends out of town all seemed to move to texting or email rather than phone calls. That caused as need for practice, but when tired the effects of slurring letters, words worsened. At first, only early in the morning or late at night when I showed general tiredness, did my speech suffer. But as I aged, I needed to be more focused on speaking clearly. When interacting with store clerks or others unfamiliar with me, I often had to repeat things two, sometimes three times. All this is just to alert the need for communicating regularly even if about simply talking sports or the weather. If not, them out loud reading of somethings every morning or a few times per week even need. to be done to keep limber, in practice. If alone even sing or try to anyway.

Tips and Notes for Improving speech and communication

.The exercises that the speech therapist would of in a hospital or outpatient care setting should be continued in the home exercises as in front of a mirror. In general, mirrors are extremely helpful in recovery in the home as being able to watch movements with face, arms or legs is so beneficial.

Communication can be improved between the injured or affected and family members by speaking short sentences and keeping concepts singular say not complicated. Speaking slowly does help yes but speaking exaggerated slowly especially out in public is kind of embarrassing so short sentences probably a better way. When speaking to the injured or affected person please speak in a normal tone of voice. Sometimes people try to exaggerate the slowness as if there is speaking to a little child and that is simply the wrong thing for effective communication.

Sometimes during the early healing and even years after during speech, words may come out in the incorrect order seeming disconnected at times as part of the healing process. Also, inappropriate language that may be used at times even when the injured person never used that kind of language before. I can tell you personally that brain training is available from some of the most respected sites online these days and I'll give you references, recommendation in later articles and website references in the appendix, can help immensely. A word of caution though with the training is that a small amount a day may be better even in segments, possibly in the morning, midday or night would be better than long sessions since fatigue can set in so easily.

Incontinence: Some people have difficulty controlling their bladder or bowel movements after brain injury. This can be controlled with options such as catheterization, utilization of incontinence pads or undergarments, and behavior strategies such as regularly timed voiding.

Sleep disturbances: Sleep problems can occur following a stroke or other brain injury. Sleep evaluations, supplemental oxygen and pharmaceutical interventions can help regulate sleep. A way that some, including me, have benefited here is from relaxation audio, guided meditation, and with physician's approval even brainwave entrainment to induce deep peaceful sleep.

Depression: Unfortunately for many people with hemiparesis, depression is a common side effect. Due to personal loss of independence and strength, feelings of sadness can quickly lead to depression. It has been common for people that have hemiparesis to be on long term antidepressant medications. Myself, avoiding medications is best if natural cure is available and in this case I feel the best course is continued relationships with friends, family and a strong faith.

Care after Brain Injury

After the onset of injury, the first course of treatment will be at the hospital. Imaging studies will examine the brain to look for trauma or dysfunction. A CT (computerized tomography) scan examines the brain structures. This imaging study will reveal an area of injury/dysfunction due to stroke or other brain injury. Other imaging studies that are typically performed include MRI (magnetic resonance imaging) and sometimes X-rays (radiographs) if there is suspicion of any fracture. The individual will receive care from nursing staff and physicians to ensure vital signs are stable and there is no risk of further injury or damage.

The main physician that will oversee the plan of care is the neurologist. Neurologists are physicians that specialize in the systems of the brain and nervous system. The neurologist will examine the function of the nervous system, identifying the area of damage to the brain and classifying extent of physical ramifications. Other physicians may be brought into the plan of care such as a cardiologist to oversee the monitoring of heart function, as well as a trauma doctor in case of injury. A physiatrist is a physician that specializes in rehabilitation. A physiatrist will oversee the care and progression during rehabilitation.

While in the hospital and at extended care, the patient will be cared for by nurses, nurse assistants, respiratory therapists, phlebotomists, nutritionists, case workers, psychologists, and (of course) physical, occupational and speech therapists. The three types of rehabilitation therapists have some overlapping roles, but three distinct specialties. The physical therapist specializes in functional movement training. The occupational therapist specializes in self-care training. The speech therapist specializes in speech and swallowing. Working with all three specialties is essential for rehabilitation progression.

During the recovery process, individuals are typically seen in a hospital setting, rehabilitation setting, home health setting and eventually outpatient clinic settings. The patient and family meet with many healthcare providers for a comprehensive rehabilitation journey. Functional independence and safety are the main factors in determining where a patient will be placed after hospitalization.

Rehabilitation – What's Available What to Expect

During the hospital stay, the individual will begin his rehabilitation process. The licensed therapist will perform an initial evaluation to determine current functional limitations and impairments. The physical and occupational therapists will examine strength, sensory response, coordination, walking, and ability to move in and out of bed and chairs, as well as the ability to dress and handle personal care tasks.

The first task that the skilled therapist will teach and assist with is the ability to get up from lying down in bed. If the individual needs assistance, the therapist will provide that assistance and note how much assistance is needed. Then, the therapist will assess and instruct in moving from sitting to standing and getting up to sit in a chair. These tasks are called transfers. Standing balance and stability is assessed to determine level of independence and risk for falling. If there is a need for use of an assistive device for mobility, the therapist will instruct the individual in use of a walker, cane or wheelchair. The main goal of the rehabilitation in the hospital setting is to determine current level of dependence, teach basic skills for mobility (getting in/out of bed, walking), and set up the appropriate treatment course upon discharge from the hospital.

After the acute care stay at the hospital, which typically lasts less than one week, most individuals move to an inpatient rehabilitation setting or a skilled nursing facility. These facilities serve to provide care for the individual's basic needs, such as getting in and out of bed, showering, dressing, nursing care and meals. In addition, the rehabilitation team will continue the care for teaching functional mobility training, as well as working to improve and restore balance and muscle strength. In the inpatient setting, the therapists help to order any necessary adaptive equipment, such as long handled reachers or ankle foot orthoses (AFOs). The stay in an inpatient setting can be anywhere from one week to several months. These facilities have nursing care, rehab care and visiting doctor oversight. The clients are provided with rooms (some private, some shared rooms) for sleeping and necessities. This setting serves as a transition point for individuals that need further care before return home. In addition, for individuals that are not able to return home, skilled nursing facilities offer long term care. In long term care, the individual is cared for by the skilled nursing team. This situation is for people that are dependent for basic needs, unable to care for themselves, and without others to care for them.

Outpatient physical therapy clinics are intended to continue rehabilitation after an individual has completed their initial rehabilitation stay after injury or stroke. Typically, individuals attend outpatient therapy sessions 2-3 days per week and complete their own exercises on non-therapy days. Outpatient therapy treatment cases are designed to further improve specific components of functional loss, and further improve safety with balance and mobility. Occupational therapy can be done in an outpatient setting, focusing on improving the use of the hand and upper extremity. In addition, outpatient occupational therapy works to improve self-care strategies. Speech therapy is often utilized in an outpatient setting to improve speech, articulation and swallowing.

Longer term rehabilitation need to continue as a primarily at home exercise program the physical therapists will recommend specific exercises. In the later sections, are included general exercises that can be performed at home for muscle weaknesses, foot drop, spasticity and more. Sure, there a different level of recovery and the point of ongoing exercise in many cases is to maintain the recovery or even partial recovery. Without ongoing exercise at home or in the gym or pool, a step back in physical condition can too easily occur. I can attest to the road back being a lot of work especially ongoing as one has ages. As I write this over 30 years after my initial hemiparesis effects, I'm going through many of the same range of motion exercises, hand therapy, stretching that I went through in my early twenties all because during the colder weather, I injured myself in the ice and snow Recovery now is again showing gains in strength and flexibility, certainly not as fast these days.

> In general, remember, an impact to one's brain through injury or illness can drastically affect cognitive performance. Thought processing can be slower, it can be difficult to concentrate or focus, and memory can deteriorate significantly. A brain injury can also have an impact on social skills. Concentration and focus, attention are primary traits or more likely developed skills that can be improved in time. In later sections and selected articles, numerous techniques are reviewed. The effectiveness of some will depend on extent of one's injuries and personal physicians would have the best specific advice. I can tell you that after my coma, counting numbers was an issue but years later studying for my engineering degree and subsequent professional career showed dramatic improvements in concentration, focus, accurate thinking speed and memory to start.

Specific rehabilitation treatment approaches include:

- Constraint induced movement therapy: This form of therapy restricts the use of the unaffected limb, forcing the patient to use the weakened part of the body. The therapist applies a mitten or sling to the unaffected arm to prevent the patient from using it. This forces the patient to use the weaker arm to perform everyday tasks. This process helps to build muscle strength, and functional coordination. It has been shown to improve nerve function and elicit new neural pathways.

- Functional Electrical Stimulation: Electric stimulation of the musculature is performed to elicit muscle contraction and make them more stable. Electric stimulation is often done at the shoulder and at the lower leg to compensate for shoulder subluxation and foot drop respectively. In addition, electric stimulation can be utilized to elicit muscle contraction for any area of paresis. The goal is to build muscle strength through artificial stimulation, in hopes of regaining control and regaining strength.

- Motor imagery and mental practice: With the therapist, the patient imagines performing a simple task such as standing up or walking. The area of the brain that controls movement for that task is stimulated, yielding new neuronal pathways.

- Virtual reality: Computer generated games and virtual experiences are now being used to practice daily tasks or movements. This simulated environment allows the patient to experience normal movement virtually. This strategy is intended to build new neuronal connections that will carry over into real improvements.

- Partial body weight support treatment: For individuals with weakness impacting their lower legs and trunk strength, partial body weight supported training is an excellent way to improve quality and tolerance for standing and walking. The therapist utilizes a body weight support harness for the patient, gradually decreasing the amount of support and increasing the amount of weight bearing through the patient's legs. This increases the physical demands of strength for the postural and leg muscles, as well as increases demands on balance. Partial body weight support can be combined with a treadmill to improve walking quality.

- Biofeedback: Biofeedback is a form of electrical therapy that is used to increase an individual's awareness of muscle control and activation. The therapist places electrodes on the skin over the affected muscle. The electrodes sense the amount of muscle activation and this is displayed on a monitor. The therapist helps the patient to elicit and control muscle activation in hopes of regaining strength or regaining functional use of a muscle group.

- Positioning: Positioning is utilized throughout a patient's care after brain injury. Because of limited strength and use of limbs, positioning is essential for joint safety and to reduce likelihood of skin breakdown. Positioning reduces muscle spasm, stiffness and pain. In addition, positioning helps to reduce likelihood of contractures in joints as well as improve efficiency and quality of breathing. The therapist will educate the patient in proper positioning strategies.

- Passive range of motion: Passive range of motion is performed by a therapist on the affected limbs of the patient. After brain injury, there is risk of developing stiff and rigid joints, which make any form of mobility very difficult. Passive range of motion helps to keep limbs limber and moving. It reduces pain and muscle spasm. Passive range of motion should be taught to caregivers to ensure carry over after completion of therapy.

- Strength training: The therapist will direct the patient through exercises to facilitate muscle contraction in the affected limbs. Depending on the strength presents, the patient may only be able to move a limb through partial range of motion, or move the limb fully against gravity and even with some resistance. The therapist will facilitate exercise to create strong muscle development and stimulate new motor control pathways.

- Neuromuscular re-education: This type of intervention focuses on retraining the control and response of the nervous and musculoskeletal system. Neuromuscular re-education focuses in improving balance, posture and coordination. This form of treatment allows for independent sitting posture, standing stability and the ability to reach for an object outside of the base of support. Of all the types of intervention, a significant amount is focused on neuromuscular re-education.

- Gait training: Gait refers to walking and ambulation. Depending on the extent of involvement in the legs, the individual will need to re-learn how to walk. The patient will utilize assistive devices, braces and external support. As strength and balance improve, many people can regain some functional walking.

- My personal example started after the coma, strengthening my core, legs, balance, weight bearing and range of motion exercises with physical therapy when still in the hospital. I was in a wheel chair mostly or in bed for the initial stretching, range of motion exercises and strengthening. Mostly using the wheelchair for me during the hospital stay except for the time in physical therapy daily, where eventually I would walk between two bars where my weight was semi-supported during an only less than 10 feet walk after some time of strengthening and stretching. This advanced to using a quad cane of 100 feet or so with therapist close by. After being released from the hospital and more at home exercises as leg lifts and stretching, I graduated to a straight cane and subsequently could go without it so. Years later, I still occasionally use the cane in crowded areas as airports or concerts. It can be useful as many others won't recognize your hemiparesis or muscle weakness but when you have the cane, often people just give a little more room and don't rush either. Believe me, it is safer to have with you at times even when you don't need to use it to support your weight.

- Wheelchair training: At some point after a stroke, most patients will utilize a wheelchair for at least a short duration. A wheelchair allows for safe mobility and significantly decreases fall risk. The wheelchair can be passively pushed by another person, but if wheelchair use is going to be long term, it is essential that the patient try to self-propel. There are many wheelchair styles, including motorized, tilt-in-space, and single arm drive chairs.

- Aquatic therapy: Aquatic therapy utilizes the properties of water to facilitate muscle strengthening, flexibility, balance and ease with walking. Buoyancy supports limb movement and water resistance builds strength.

Equipment

Over the course of care after an individual acquires hemiparesis, many types of equipment will be introduced. Some equipment is familiar, like a cane. Other pieces of equipment are new and others are modifications to everyday objects.

Equipment used for mobility:

- Wheelchair: A wheelchair is used for individuals that are unable to walk, or are unstable walking. The wheelchair has push handles and leg rests so that someone else can dependently push the affected individual. Wheelchairs collapse so that they can be put into vehicles and transported. There are many unique options and adaptations for wheelchairs so that it can be customized to the needs of everyone. For example, a single-arm drive wheelchair allows for self-propelling of the wheelchair with only one arm. In addition, many individuals utilize an arm support attachment for the weak or spastic affected arm.
- Walker: For individuals with weakness in one arm, a platform support can be attached to a walker. This supports the affected arm while maintaining the function of the walker.
- Hemi-walker: This mobility device is something that combines the stability of a walker with the small size of a cane. The hemi walker is held by the strong arm and has a wide base of support on the ground. It is used in walking sequence just like a cane.
- Quad cane: There are two variations of a quad cane, a small base quad cane and large base quad cane. This cane has four contact points (quad) and provides greater support in comparison to a traditional single point cane.
- Single point cane: This cane has one single point and provides the least amount of support.
- Slide board: A slide board is a board that is used to complete a transfer from one seated surface to another. For example: a slide board is commonly used to transfer an individual from bed to a wheelchair. The board is placed

under the individual's bottom, bridging the space between one chair to the other chair. The individuals "slides" across the slide board (usually with assistance from a caregiver). The slide board is intended for individuals that cannot safely bear weight through their legs to transfer.

- Hoyer lift: This is a mechanical lift that is intended for individuals that are dependent for mobility. The individual is lifted by the machine, enclosed in a support sling. This keeps that patient safe and eliminates physical strain for the caregiver.
- Standing lift: For individuals that can tolerate standing position, but are unable to come to standing, the standing lift assists in transfers. The patient is supported by a sling, and the feet are positioned on a standing plate. The machine lifts the patient to stand and supports them in that position.
- Orthotics: If there is persistent inability to lift the toe for walking or weakness around the foot and lower leg, an orthotic may be required. An ankle foot orthosis serves to control impaired ankle/foot function and allow for improved walking.

Self-care equipment:

- Long handled reacher: A reacher is a long pole with a grabber at the end. It is intended to help grab clothing and other daily items when an individual does not have the strength or balance to reach for an item otherwise.
- Sock aid: A sock aid is a commonly used device that aids in putting on socks. It is used by placing the sock over the rounded, half circle device and then sliding the sock right over the foot.
- Adaptive utensils: For individuals with involvement at the hand, it can be difficult to use utensils for eating. For this reason, there are knives designed with a rocker handle to

allow for easier cutting. In addition, there are wide grip forks and spoons to allow for easier holding and grasp.

- Shower chair/bench: For bathing, many individuals do not have the strength or balance to take a shower standing upright. Shower chairs and shower benches create a safer environment for personal hygiene. The individual sits on the shower bench and uses a hand-held showerhead for washing.
- Raised toilet seats: Standing up from a low toilet seat can be very difficult for people with hemiparesis. Therefore, adaptations can be made with a raised toilet seat to allow for easier transfers from the toilet.
- Adjustable Toilet Safety Rails – The height and width are adjustable in these for stability and leverage when standing. Also sitting down gradually as to avoid and impact is also aided greatly when using this option.
- Re Toilet seat adjustments – These assistive devices or aids mentioned here are great in the home but won't help when traveling or even out to a local restaurant. A handicapped toilet is not always readily available. I can't recommend enough in this book to keep the weight off and stretch regularly to keep flexible.
- Grab bars: Grab bars are vital for safety in the bathroom. They should be placed next to the toilet and in and around the shower. Grab bars must be installed into the studs of the wall to ensure proper support and anchoring.
- Shower Slippers – These allow feet to be washed while being worn as these are made of a breathable weave. The result is more confident footing

Bathroom Care and Shower Safety

Safety in the shower and bath deserves its own section and I cannot emphasize the importance of it enough. Outlined are some key considerations but also contained in this chapter are insights from the authors experience of the last three decades. The authors insights are mostly for the affected person experiencing the balance issues, possible slippage, potential awkward sudden movements.

Shower Considerations

If possible, a walk-in shower is safest and easiest to use. And next a shower and select preferred than bathtubs. With a weakened side, it can be terribly awkward to enter and especially leave what can be a slippery surface. The shower is also easier for your family to assist you in or out while possibly having to lift you out of a tub. A crucial point is that many of us do not have family living with us that can assist, and in addition it should be strongly noted that help is not always wanted, only reluctantly being asked for. Sometimes, the need for independent living overlooks proper safety, but independence and safety should be considered equally.

The author's experience with hemiparesis living has proven that there are both inexpensive safety precautions and free advice that is invaluable when considering bathroom and shower safety. Listed next, is an outline of safety and care items followed by more detail added from personal experience as advisement on issues that arise day to day that if not prepared for, can cause injury to the affected. It may seem like too much detail in areas but for the injured. On the other hand, for family members or care taker, reading through the important points outlined, bolded for a faster read should suffice.

Before entering the shower, itself,

The bathroom floor is an area of concern for safety. Earlier I had mentioned the throw rugs throughout the house could be removed as a safety precaution. However, many bathroom floors are made of a tile, ceramic or polished wood and can be super slick especially for person with a weakened foot or drop foot condition. In this case I do recommend a large rug but it must have rubber backing and be adhered to the floor in some way. To do this, there are several good systems available at your local hardware store even as simple as double-faced tape. Of course, if you have wall-to-wall carpet in the bath or self-adhering carpet tiles, this is a nonissue.

Tips For the actual shower.

A first consideration should be grab bars. For your home, these can be screwed into the wall as the safest measure how. However, hardware stores are now selling the suction cup plastic grab bars in a variety of sizes and shapes. I've used these plastic grab bars myself in apartments I lived in and currently use them. I strongly must recommend a redundant system though, as these are economical enough to have multiple grab bars within the shower.

Exiting the shower is dangerous especially in these cases when you land on the foot drop affected side. At some point the better leg is lifted off the ground entering or exiting leaving the affected foot bearing the weight plus the good and grasping the grab bar. Since the affected foot when bare has no or little friction or grab to the floor, the location of entering and exiting should have a short 8-12-inch grab bar or even two located preferably vertically. I recommend two if you are using the suction cups so that you have a redundant system that is safer.

In the shower space, needs to be located a larger horizontal grab bar. Many showers these days have one built in as part of the enclosure. The crucial point is that the person should be able to easily grab a bar with their better hand from anywhere they may stand. If they are using a shower seat. or a bench that is part of the enclosure itself

The shower or bath mat is another primary concern. It should be large, even oversize that has a gripper. If the drain hole is in the center of the shower, make sure the mat allows water to run right through it. If not water permeable when having a center drain hole in a shower, water collects on the surface, mat can become soggy and bunch up under feet. I've experienced my foot in this unsafe condition and am thankful for the grab bars when this occurred.

Important added notes showers and on the use of suction cup secured grab bars.

While the secured to the wall grab bars are recommended, the grab bars that are available with strong suction cups are also used. These are valuable for apartment dwellers or travelers where secured grab bars are not always available or able to install as desired. When using them however, as a safety precaution, before entering the shower, when dry, tap the grab bars lightly to check whether they are secure and if not adjust them so that they are.

I can tell you from experience that one of the worst things that can happen in the shower is for someone as myself with a weakened side to reach out with your strong hand for something to grasp onto and have it just fall onto the floor shower. Usually when you reach out for something to grasp, that is a time when there may have soap in your eye or worse possibly losing your balance and slipping. These are the times that are critical to one's safety and why having taken the time taken to make sure the grab bars are secure when entering is invaluable.

Please take these safety tips seriously in the bath and shower from one who has fallen and seriously injured myself.

It can happen so fast. Even after years of successfully entering, exiting and showering, the safety concern is still just as important. **Often showers are taken early in the morning or late at night when tired.** This is a crucial point as it is when we are tired that the worst detrimental effects are exhibited. The sudden dragging of the foot or a sudden loss in balance because the affected foot lands on the side or at an angle rather than flat on the heel or soles of a foot. When tired, balance can be effected more. I can attest to leaning backwards more often and reaching out for something to hold onto. If this feeling of falling backwards occurs in the shower or even when shaving, it leads to awkward reaching out for something stable to hang onto. And in the case of falling backwards, for hemiparesis affected, this is real not imaginary. It is mostly unpredictable but there are occasions where it may occur more. In the bath or shower room, when tired after waking or before bed, was when this uneasiness feeing occurred for me and several times where falling was prevented because of a clean well equipped with grab bars in several locations.

Movements During a Shower

Soaping and cleaning under the affected weaker arm can be accomplished easier by leaning forward slightly. This could cause a balance issue in the shower and recommended instead is a hand-held shower head with hose that is attached to fixture shower head. Also, a long-handled brush will assist under the arms and prevent any reaching or bending over. Scrub pals are name brand extended handled brushes that come in several shapes, nine and 17 inch lengths. Of course, a search on the Internet or your local home and body shop will provide many options.

If you do have to bend over for dropped soap or shampoo bottle, think out everything you must do to retrieve it. I know this sounds simple but any sudden move can be disastrous in a shower when you need your stronger hand to hold on when bending over and then also to pick the item up. Kind of a situation that could be unsafe if not planned One method is to have your stronger side close to the shower wall, hold a fixed bar as you bend over for the soap or item, then, just before you let go of the support bar, make sure both feet are in the direction of the item so that you will not be twisting when you pick up item. After letting go of the bar, pick up item slowly and place on a ledge or shower bench if one is there. Then grab the bar again with your stronger hand and when grasping bar and feet stable rise out of the bent position. Really breaking down he movement but trust me on this, you absolutely need to take the extra precautions in the shower area.

Of course, having extra soaps in a basket suctioned to the wall about waste high plus extra shampoo would be ideal. Retrieving the items later in a dry shower would be safest.

There also are extender grab hands that are available. Shower slippers are available for more confident footing. They allow fee to be washed while being worn as they are made of a breathable weave.

Shaving in the Bathroom

The obvious first choice would be to use an electric shaver if possible. However, some people cannot due to pain on the affected side. Some as myself still prefer the close shave of a blade but just can't use a straight razor safely. Well a straight razor is not a choice with me as I also had the tips of my fingers affected from nerve injury in an accident. The best compromise for years was the multiple blade shavers that were a step safer than the single blade. Now electric shavers have improved immensely and even offer wet shaving. I feel that the wet shave could give the closest shave for a safe way to shave. Note that applying shaving cream could be easiest by using an aerosol can of shaving cream pointed at the top of the weakened hand and then using the stronger hand to scoop up and apply to face. Some of the wet shavers can be put right under the faucet too for rinsing which does help speed this process. For hemiparesis survivors, an important safety concern is standing and balance of course. Leaning backwards or to the weakened side is another concern long term.

Allow for extra time here as men will need to spend extra care and time on the affected side of his face depending on extent on injury or illness. Women too should plan for extra time and care under their weakened arm and for their legs.

Final Note on Showering

My experience has enabled me to just assure the key safety items and habits or processes are followed. This was never more important since the early years after 'acquiring' the one side weakness or partial paralysis, plus about a ten-year span later spent living successfully alone.   Safety in everyday activities especially in your own home as bath and shower simply cannot get enough detail because of safety.

Exercise Ongoing After Therapy Services

Despite rehabilitation efforts, many individuals do not regain full strength, balance and independence. After therapy services have been discontinued, it is essential that people continue exercising on their own.

Land exercise: There are many limitations that should be addressed through exercise for optimal mobility and pain relief. It is important to keep full range of motion in the affected limb or limbs. For many people, spasticity limits how well a joint can fully bend or straighten. Active range of motion exercises are those in which the individual moves the arm fully straight and then fully bent. These simple exercises keep the joints limber and moving.

Strengthening exercises - It is also important to keep up with strengthening exercises. Strengthening exercises should be done for the entire body, not only the affected limb. The unaffected side of the body needs to compensate for weakness on the involved side. Therefore, both sides of the body need strengthening to support functional movement.

Balance training should be performed in a safe environment, such as with a caregiver or loved one. This is because people that have hemiparesis have a higher risk of falling and injury. To challenge balance, sit or stand without any upper body support. Then, practice standing with feet together and reaching forward. It is important to have a counter or chair available for purposes of grabbing to avoid falling.

Cardiovascular exercise should be incorporated to promote healthy heart and lung function. Unfortunately, for many people with hemiparesis, endurance is low and the heart and lungs do not tolerate a lot of activity. Walking, cycling, and other cardiovascular machines are great ways to improve endurance. The NuStep is a seated stepping machine that incorporates arm and leg movement and is an excellent and safe option for individuals with hemiparesis.

Aquatic exercise: Exercising in water is an excellent way to improve strength, endurance and flexibility. By choosing the right pool, you can exercise while reducing joint pain as well. Warm water pools promote improved muscular flexibility, while cool water pools help reduce swelling or edema in limbs. Water has properties of buoyancy and resistance, which can be used to build muscle and alleviate pain.

The buoyancy of water allows for joint decompression while submerged. The water buoyancy supports your limbs in a way that is not experienced while on land. It is as if there is an artificial brace around your joints or spine. This is excellent for individuals that have joint pain after onset of hemiparesis. Because of the buoyancy of water, most people have little pain while exercising in the pool. This phenomenon allows people to more fully participate in the exercise to improve cardiovascular endurance and muscle strength.

Water also resists movement. Resistance allows people to perform strength training in the water. When a limb is moved up and down or back and forth under the water, it must fight against the water's resistance. This strengthens the musculature. Greater resistance is elicited by using a broad paddle or board and pushing it through the water. Moving the limbs quickly also increases the resistance and engages abdominal strengthening.

Walking in water is a great form of exercise, as it simulates walking on land, but in a supportive medium. Traditional swimming is excellent for building cardiovascular endurance. Stretching in a warm water pool, promotes improved muscle flexibility and allows for stretching of tight joints. Many aquatic centers have classes that are meant for individuals with hemiparesis, which may be a terrific way to start getting into aquatic exercise.

Brain Training –

Cognitive problems can be similar after a stroke or a head injury. Common traits as brain fog, the inability to follow conversations, memory issues, comprehension even in short term reading and not being able to recall what one just read.

Not all people develop the same symptoms, but common symptoms depending on severity of injury can include confusion, headaches, irritability, nausea, blurred vision, difficulties with body balance, fatigue, slurred speech, lightheadedness, noise or light sensitivity, lack of concentration, memory disturbances, sleep disturbances, alterations in your normal sense of taste and ringing in your ears.

. Part of the goal at the early stage in rehabilitation is continued restoration of your previous skills and abilities. However, not all brain injury patients can regain normal function, and another goal of rehabilitation is teaching you how to adjust and adapt in the face of permanent changes in your physical and/or mental skill set.

Experts have proven that the brain is able to keep learning and changing regardless of its age. This means that what you have done up to this point, you can make your brains activity better than ever.

Signs that may likely occur to different degrees as finding it difficult to pay attention to things going on around oneself. Also reading or listening to information and then being unable to recall any of the details when finished. The brain is having difficulty staying focused on what you're doing.

By engaging in a variety of exercises for your brain you will learn to focus your attention. This is a very valuable skill that will be used in all aspects of your life. It can be hard when you begin, as some become frustrated and quit. Keep reminding yourself of what will be accomplished once you've cleared the hurdles standing in your way.

When I came home from the hospital in my twenties, one of the first activities that I had was just trying some of the puzzle books and magazines that were for my daughter. Now my daughter at that time wasn't even old enough for kindergarten. These simple games for the brain that were designed for preschoolers were very good for me. They tired me out after a short while at first just minutes, then a half hour, then more. I graduated to an electronic game that you can get at many stores even online at Amazon. Of course, they have everything there. But anyway, the game Brain Age in this Nintendo game had a quiz that tested your brain age. They have many more these days after the popularity of Brain Age, but Brain Age remains a great start. It worked on how fast and well you answered questions, simple memory tests and quizzes and even calculations if you were interested in that. You can choose the type of questions. My age showed me that my brain was that of a 76-year-old! Wow, for me in my mid-twenties that was eye opening. I used the games on Brain Age daily, 5 to 10 minutes a day, sometimes more for quite some time. I tested myself monthly and most months I improved my brain age until it was very close to my real age. I reduced it to 30 eventually

My speed of thinking improved and I graduated to online exercises for brain training. One site that has various levels from beginning to expert plus allows you to compare yourself against different age groups is Lumosity.com.

As you work on exercising your brain you will start to see an improvement in your processing speed. You will find that you are completing certain tasks more quickly. You will start to comprehend things you have read the first time and will no longer have to read everything two or three times. Things that caused you to struggle in the past will start to be very clear; it will feel like someone has flipped a switch inside you.

More advanced is BrainHQ.com - When it comes to brain fitness training, BrainHQ is **best in class**. Built by a **team of top neuroscientists**, with **exercises proven in dozens of published studies** to make real and lasting improvements in brain function, BrainHQ is your personal brain gym.

The real proof was how I felt listening and talking to others. My communication improved, my thinking was better with better memory too. I even enrolled in summer classes at a State University to test my brain competing with some very bright students and did very well with a B in my first class.

It is very important to exercise your brain so that you will be able to keep these benefits. If you don't want to lose the skills you have, you will have to keep them sharp. Make it a priority to continue learning all the things in the world as you grow older. If there are things you want to explore, make a list of them. Discover ways to learn these things while exercising your brain and you will get twice the benefits from your efforts.

Before long, you will start to notice some very significant changes to your thought process. You will process information more quickly, remember more, and you will have no problem focusing your attention where you need to. Your life will become more enjoyable no matter what you take part in.

Now that you know more about the incredible benefits of exercising your brain, find some activities to take part in that will keep your mind healthy. Of course, an injury to the brain can have limited success from simply exercising it, with usage but advances are still occurring and brain recovery is amazing. Brain training even after injury or illness through knowledge of plasticity and a better definition of audio software effects especially the last couple decades and it's all good news for us You can do even many of them alone at home or play games online. There are many that you can do with someone else too. The key is to find plenty of brain exercises that you find intriguing. Then make a commitment to do them often. If some do not have effects you desire, others may. Remain positive.

Brain Training Online –

This book's focus is at home care, rehabilitation and exercise so continuing with this, brain training online can gradually improve brain function as the specific targeted brain training exercises that can start at an easy level, then get progressively more difficult spurring growth in the brain.

To show a significant noticeable improvement, recommended is daily brain training for 6 to 8 weeks. Starting with a ten to twenty-minute session, preferably an hour a day may need to be worked up to. Some persons focus and concentration just need to be worked up to. I can tell you that with the auditory training from brainHQ.com mentioned, I was able to listen better and understand other people's communication. This was in unexpected bonus from the training to me anyway, the concentration and focus improved noticeably after only a few days.

Even after years, improvement can be gained, but we need to work at it. BrainHQ has a "Brain Injury Survivor" Set of Exercises proven to improve auditory processing, memory, people skills, focusing one's attention. Also, to improve the brain's ability to pay attention, especially in difficult conditions. They help you stay on task even when you need to keep track of many things at once or spot subtle details. Visit, http://brainhq.com to try free.

The internet does have some websites of value and the brain training available is improving drastically. I will provide additional resources in the appendix and at one of my own websites http://hemiparesisliving.com/helpful-resources/

Brain Training through Meditation

Another daily practice that improves anyone's mind is meditation in the mornings. This ancient practice of meditation still may be the best exercise or practice that can transform the structure of your brain and mental thought patterns. A type recommended is specifically mindfulness meditation. I'm including a couple of my published articles in the appendix for beginning meditation practices. Mindfulness meditation can be done anywhere to find a quiet place makes it easier when you first begin. I've also included a mindfulness meditation for beginning article in the appendix.

Focus and Concentration are the Key - From the start of rehabilitation exercises, though walking keeping your arm straight, your leg straight, taking notice of how your foot lands to more advanced at home skills as in the kitchen with knives or the oven, to even driving on the interstate all require the survivor to concentrate strongly for them anyway. Sure, these activities may seem either natural for most or insignificant to most people but to the head injured or stroke survivors living with hemiparesis there is a "re-learning" curve. Fortunately, brain plasticity allows some functions to return as "second nature". Not all, of course as for many tasks ranging from simple walking to showering need a consistent focused attention to stay safe first and avoid accidents.

Focus is essential to all cognitive tasks. The ability to sustain attention amidst external distractions aids greatly in the ability of the brain to take on new mental challenges Focus is essential to all cognitive tasks. The ability to sustain attention amidst external distractions aids greatly in the ability of the brain to take on new mental challenges

I state this as in the articles I'll add later in the book on improving your mind, thinking ability. memory, focus and concentration, ability to think clearly, decision making, or other, I did not limit most of these in any way as if to imply a damaged brain would have limitations. It may have of course on an individual basis and in some cases extremely limited. People vary greatly with intellect before either their injuries or stroke and certainly the degree of how far they return to former brain processing levels or even excel further. If there are indeed limitations individually, that is between you and your physicians. I present most of the brain improvement articles as what can be achieved. Certainly, there will be limitations but it is note within the scope of this book to distinguish the many levels of recovery. Myself, I've had a successful engineering career. I know nurses and lawyers too that have gone through either a traumatic brain injury or a stroke of varying degrees. Even as all mentioned still have physical limitations and some mental, they have achieved a high degree of professional achievement. We have been blessed in our recoveries for others achieving strong personal relationships with their families and friends is their first preference. Either way the basics of cognitive improvement remain the same. Some will focus more on developing communication skills rather than analytical. But the ability to focus well remains and essential characteristic of success.

Impact on Daily Life

With hemiparesis, daily life is obviously affected. Exercise at home and assistive aids will help to increase mobility and improve independence. Repeated practice of regular daily activity increases body control and coordination for daily tasks. Individuals with hemiparesis learn to perform daily tasks in a modified manner and with compensatory adaptations.

- Driving: It is essential to participate in a driving program after rehabilitation, if the individuals plans to return to driving. Eyesight, cognition and reaction time are evaluated to determine safety while driving. Even if the individual has weakness in the right leg, vehicles can be modified with hand controls for independent driving Use of a spinner knob allows ease of parking and being able to get out of situation easily and safety. In some states, you may need a doctor's approval to get one installed. In other states, they sell these over the counter at auto part stores. I would opt for the professional installation with these and the sturdier it is, the better. Don't skimp when it comes to safety in a vehicle.

- Dressing: Use of adaptive aids such as a sock aid and a reacher allow many individuals to continue dressing themselves independently. With adaptive clothing using snap closures, Velcro instead of buttons dressing is easier. The even have pans that can be changed from a seating position completely. Button down shirts can be challenging, but can be successfully performed with a buttoning aid. There are many adaptive aids available such as side opening pans, zipper front dresses or robes, custom design shoes for drop foot and Velcro closures. Myself I must laugh sometimes but I feel it necessary to have a bib during eating at times and none-skid socks around the home. It is difficult to find clothing under searches for hemiparesis living but regardless of how this illness or injury occurred, searching for stroke patient clothing and adaptation will give you a wide availability of suppliers. Silvert.com is recommended not only for the large line of specialty clothing available for men and women but also for valuable information on how one with limited movement should dress and videos free online with tips for dressing.
- Kitchen: Adaptations can be made to the countertops and cabinets to allow for wheelchair access, if needed. Regularly used items should be stored within easy reach. Meal preparation can be more challenging with hemiparesis, but adaptive utensils make this easier. Microwave use can be safer than stovetop for individuals with any cognitive impairment. Use. Lightweight non – breakable dishes. Moving food around might be better when using a rolling cart. Sliding items along a countertop or moving them short distances without moving your feet is often the smart way to go to prevent spills or dropping an item.

- Communication issues: Depending on the part of the brain affected, it may be difficult to express or understand others verbally. Utilization of alternate forms of communication can compensate for limited verbal communication. Gestures, demonstration, communication boards and reading and writing are viable options for communication difficulties.
- Working with hemiparesis: Even with weakness on one side of the body, many people go on to live very productive lives through work, social and recreational activities. Because of improvements to laws in the United States, employers cannot discriminate against individual's due to disability. Employers can make reasonable accommodations for equipment space to allow for continued work. For many individuals, cognition is not impaired, therefore critical thinking is not affected. Therefore, physical disabilities should not limit access to meaningful occupation.

Overview of Living with Hemiparesis and Safety

Safety would be the primary concern of course when people with hemiparesis live alone or are alone for extended amounts of time. Of course, your first references are your doctor, physical therapist and occupational therapists especially. This being stated, I can offer insights on some important items to consider in practical aspects of living alone after a traumatic brain injury or a stroke that result in a severe muscle weakness along the left or right side of the body and is sometimes exhibited in slight nerve damage as with me. Perhaps instead of living by themselves, it would be better to consider us living independently. At this writing, I will have reached almost thirty years of living with hemiparesis. Most of this time I was living alone and working as an engineer and writer, author.

For us, the detrimental effects of hemiparesis are still prevalent even after initial rehabilitation and limited recovery. The effects can change with extreme variation.

Effects When Tired or Awoken

When the body is tired, effects can be worse and certainly more dangerous when living alone. An example is if awoken in the night, maybe by thirst, a call, or other concern. Even a healthy person could possibly stumble on sleepy legs or with eyes half open, but for those with left or right hemiparesis, the negative effects are magnified. A stumble can turn into a fall and possibly a head injury since one arm has poor strength, does not react quickly and is not likely to stop a fall. If a foot drags slightly during the day with shoes, then it can be so much worse at night even so unsafe that the person will roll over the toes to bruise them and fall forward on the weak side. Lessons learned here emphasize the need for uncluttered floors and hallways. A stray shoe on the floor or even newspaper can prove disastrous. Either could throw off the balance suddenly for a waking person especially in the dark.

This brings up a suggestion for low level lighting in the home or apartment. Economical battery-operated motion detector lights are available at many stores now or a search online. Even if a cane is not needed during the day; it would be wise to have a cane near the bed, even a quad cane for late night awakenings or an early morning rising. In the morning, there are other issues as tightened up leg muscles that need stretching before safely moving.

Shower and Bathroom Safety

Morning stretching is important, especially as we who are injured age but more importantly, shower safety needs to be addressed. There are much assistive devices available and occupational therapists can communicate effectively the needs here, however I can give you my thoughts. These are that it can be quite scary at times, especially if you have had an accident, falling in the shower, tub or bathroom before. You will need to be able to have something within reach on your good side to grab onto, basically always. Please note that if you can't use the screwed in support rails and use the bars with suction cups, you really need at least two bars together. Redundant support as these are known to slip and when you have water or soap in your eyes and reach out with the bar slipping, it can be devastating. I would recommend having a bar on the entry or exit and on the opposite side. This way if a person with hemiparesis turns around there is always a bar on the good side.

But it does not stop there. Bathroom floors are usually smooth surfaces and with one foot having no or minimal grab, then any water on a smooth tile or marble surface is like ice and can easily cause a fall when drying. Rubber backed rugs are most often used but can bunch up under feet. A work around solution for these throw rugs is rubber strips with adhesive on both sides. The local hardware store will have some rug grippers or search the web

Dressing

This is an area again where an occupational therapist assures you are prepared with any assistive devices for reaching around the weak side or fastening in back and collar. However, I can emphasize that so much more time needs to be available, just in case. Even though, there are assistive devices and there is ample training in doing this usually available before even leaving the hospital.

Food Preparation, Cooking Kitchen Safety

One's ability to prepare meals will vary. I understand it's good to be independent but in the kitchen, it just may be smarter to minimize preparation with knives or stovetop. Even the oven can cause burns and fire easily. Having a cardboard pizza box fall onto a hot broiler iron can start a fire that is not too easy for someone with a disability to put out quickly. Sure, there are now small convenient fire extinguishers available but some often need two capable hands to operate correctly and then even finding it quickly can be an issue for trauma, brain injury or stroke victims.

Fortunately, there has been an improvement in microwave dinners. This certainly would not be your first option in the past. However, I have been at this for over thirty years now and I really have seen a wide variety come on the market and costs go down. Good, healthy dinners can be cooked in one minute. I still bake chicken and pizza plus a few others but safety really needs to be the priority. Losing balance and reaching out to find as hot frying pan to lean on can happen and I have personal experience, it's not a quick heal having a burn in the palm of your good hand. Again, here as in the bathroom, a rug with rubber backing and rug grabbers should be required.

Mind Body Health Needs

Concentration and Focus are the key in most everything that the person with hemiparesis might have to overcome. That is why ongoing brain training is so important.

Human interaction, relationships contribute greatly to complex usage of our brain and even helping to stay young. Well living alone minimizes this benefit ad over time can have an adverse effect. Sure, some will say the upward potential may be limited but start with the objective of not losing ability. Without regular exercise, mind or body can atrophy to borrow a term used to describe not using muscles.

There are free and paid sources on the web. There are now brain improvement magazines at the local supermarket and brain games are popular and effective, most even for one hand use.

Geographic Area Specific Issues

Depending on your locality, power outages can occur during natural events mostly as snow or ice storms, hurricanes, tornadoes. When living on the eastern coast, I lost power even when there was a high windstorm. Natural events as this can have an impact on people living with hemiparesis just as they do for others with a disability, elderly or families in general. However, preparedness is the key here and living alone increases importance of having battery lighting, food, water, cell phone, radio, all available and easily attainable in possibly in the dark.

The power loss may be worse in freezing weather for this condition as detrimental effects can disable some people with this extreme muscle weakness and possibly nerve damage. This varies of course depending on person or injury but in general arms and legs can start shaking uncontrollably and a serious limitation to mobility. Poor effects are also exhibit in sudden changes of weather. Each person may experience this differently but a check with your physician is best.

To assist in times as these, warm clothing, even a safe generator where it can be installed in a home as a backup are suggestions with heat packs available at sporting goods stores or camping supply shop.

Summary

Some of the techniques and tips outlined here may seem obvious to some or simple but they are not always thought of ahead of time before they are used. This is evident in support forums online, knowing individuals and my own thirty years of living with hemiparesis. There are of course more but in general, consideration that movements can be slow at times as can thinking. A key point is if there is a loss of balance or tripping, it will most likely be on the weak side which of course doesn't react fast nor have enough hand strength usually to hang on to something firmly. Therefore, safety is the priority when living alone with this injury.

The condition of foot drop has a significant impact for the person living with hemiparesis There is a separate chapter on the issues care and rehabilitation of foot drop that follows.

Foot Drop Condition, Care, Rehabilitation Exercises and Safety

What is Foot Drop?

Foot drop is a paralysis or weakness of muscles that causes difficulty in lifting the forefoot. This leads to an abnormal walking pattern, with the forefoot dragging along the ground. People with foot drop often compensate by lifting the knee higher while walking.

Foot drop is not a medical condition. Instead, it is a symptom of an underlying problem. Conditions that cause nerve damage, systemic muscular weakness or injury to the spine can all cause foot drop.

Symptoms of Foot Drop

A person with foot drop finds it difficult or impossible to lift the front of their foot. This causes the foot to drag along the ground during a normal gait pattern.

To stop the foot hitting the ground, people with foot drop develop an abnormal gait. Common abnormalities include lifting the hip, to provide more clearance, and swinging the leg out to the side.

Diagnosis of foot drop can take place during a physical examination by a doctor. Once foot drop has been diagnosed, it is important to find the underlying cause. If there is no obvious source of foot drop, medical imaging techniques such as CT scans, X-rays or ultrasound scans may be recommended. In some cases, tests to find nerve damage are also required.

Causes of Foot Drop

Any condition that causes muscular weakness or nerve damage can potentially cause foot drop. Drop foot may also be a symptom of a neurological disease such as multiple sclerosis, or conditions such as cerebral palsy and a stroke.

Muscular Weakness

The muscles of the lower leg that pull the ankle and foot up are called dorsiflexors. If these muscles are weak or inhibited, they cannot provide the required force to lift the foot up fully, leading to foot drop. This weakness can be caused by conditions such as spinal muscular atrophy, motor neuron disease and muscular dystrophy.

Nerve Damage

Each muscle is controlled, or innervated, by a nerve that tells the muscle when to contract or relax. The dorsiflexors are innervated by the peroneal nerve. If this nerve, or any leading to it, become trapped or damaged, electrical signals telling the muscles to contract may not get through. This can result in drop foot.

Damage to the nerves that control the ankle dorsiflexors can occur through a traumatic accident, injury during surgery or because of conditions affecting the nerves. Nerve damage from diabetes can also cause foot drop.

Treatments and Management

The most effective treatments for foot drop depend on the underlying cause. The earlier treatment begins – especially with physical therapy – the greater chance of significant improvement in function.

Braces (Ankle-foot Orthotics)

Braces, or ankle-foot orthotics (AFO), are often used to minimize the effects of drop foot. The braces are lightweight and usually support the ankle at 90 degrees. There are other types of braces which allow more movement, depending on the patient's level of function. It's important to wear a tight-fitting sock while using a brace to prevent excessive rubbing.

A brace may be used temporarily, until other treatments have improved the condition, or permanently. For permanent foot drop, a custom brace is often built for more comfortable long-term use. The lightest braces are made of plastic or carbon, while heavier models are built from leather or metal. Plastic is often the material used for custom orthotics, as it can be molded to the patient's dimensions.

Some people with foot drop find that a brace helps them to walk more normally. Others find a brace uncomfortable or think that a brace is unsightly with certain types of clothing. For many patients with foot drop, the long-term goal is to avoid using an AFO. While this may be possible, it is important that a brace is used until the patient's healthcare professional indicates it is no longer required.

Physical Therapy

Physical therapy can potentially lead to a partial or full recovery from foot drop. The long-term outcome depends on the underlying cause and how quickly the person receives treatment. A patient with some ability to move the foot when first visiting a physical therapist is more likely to achieve greater improvement.

A physical therapist will create an individual program for each patient. This program may contain a variety of types of exercises, including:

> Strengthening Exercises. If the muscles of the leg and foot become stronger, a person with drop foot may find it easier to walk normally. Strengthening exercises also prevent or delay muscles from becoming progressively weaker.
>
> Stretching Exercises. It's important that a person with foot drop actively stretches to maintain muscle length. This helps prevent restricted range of motion in the ankle and knee.
>
> Gait Training. If a patient has developed an abnormal gait pattern, a physical therapist can re-train him or her to use a safer pattern. Gait training is also important after surgery.

Balance Exercises. Some patients with foot drop find it difficult to walk on uneven surfaces. A physical therapist may re-teach the patient how to walk on surfaces such as sand or bumpy ground.

A later section of this report provides an overview of the most common physical therapy exercises for drop foot.

Functional Electrical Stimulation

Functional electrical stimulation, more commonly known as FES, involves applying electrical currents to a nerve that isn't receiving the correct signals from the brain or spine. By applying a current to the peroneal nerve, for example, the muscles at the front of the ankle can be contracted during the gait cycle. Sensors are placed in the heel of the shoe to sense when the muscles need to be activated. FES can promote a more normal gait pattern.

FES has a number of benefits compared to braces. The devices are much smaller and work with regular shoes. In some cases, FES also helps to improve nerve function. The downside is the cost – FES devices are far more expensive than ankle-foot orthotics.

While this type of treatment can be effective for drop foot, it is not suitable for everyone. FES is most effective for foot drop caused by damage or injury to the brain or spinal cord. FES is not a cure for foot drop, but can minimize its effect on everyday life.

Surgery

Surgery for foot drop may be appropriate to resolve certain underlying conditions. If a nerve is damaged or trapped, for example, surgery to decompress the nerve could potentially lead to a recovery in function. For foot drop caused by a herniated disc in the spine, which can press on the nerve controlling muscles in the leg, surgery can also be effective.

If foot drop is permanent, a doctor may recommend surgery to fuse the ankle bones. This provides more stability and can make walking easier. Another common type of surgery for foot drop involves transferring a tendon from a different muscle to improve ankle stability.

Caring for Foot Drop at Home

Foot drop can be temporary or permanent, and may affect one or both feet. A person with foot drop may need to make lifestyle adjustments for increased safety and management of the problem.

Home Exercises

A patient with foot drop will typically have one or two sessions with a physical therapist each week. These sessions alone usually aren't enough to achieve significant improvement. For this reason, a physical therapist will create a home exercise program. Following this program is vital for managing and improving foot drop.

Emotional Support

Foot drop can be emotionally distressing. There may be activities or daily tasks that become much more difficult for the patient. For this reason, the support of medical professionals, family, and friends in the patient's home is an important part of coping with foot drop.

Pain Management

Foot drop may be painful depending on the underlying condition. It is important to manage the pain to prevent it from getting progressively worse. The patient should discuss pain management options with his or her doctor.

Safety

A person with foot drop has an increased risk of falling over. This risk can be reduced by being careful when walking and by using a brace. Some people with foot drop also find it useful to use a walking stick. A stick can be especially useful when walking in crowded areas.

It's important to remove any potentially dangerous obstacles from the home. Other family members should be aware of items or clutter that could be dangerous and move them off the floor whenever possible. Rugs, in particular, can be a slipping hazard. It is also a clever idea to remove any electrical cords that are close to walkways.

Every case of foot drop needs to be evaluated individually to judge the safety of certain activities. Many people with foot drop stay active, although walking can become tiring more quickly. The level of safe activity depends on the severity of foot drop and the underlying condition.

Exercises for foot drop

A physical therapist may prescribe a range of exercises to maintain joint motion, increase muscle strength and improve ankle stability. Some of the most common exercises include:

Calf Stretch. The patient sits with legs out in-front. Placing a towel around the toes of the foot, the patient gently pulls the forefoot towards the body. This provides a stretch to the calf muscles and prevents a loss of joint mobility.

Toe Curls. Start by placing a rolled-up towel on the floor. While sitting, the patient curls the toes of the affected foot to scrunch up the towel.

Straight Leg Raises. The patient lies on the floor with upper body propped up on elbows and one leg bent. He or she then contracts the quadriceps (upper thigh muscles) of the straight leg and slowly lifts the leg off the floor until it is at the height of the bent knee. This exercise strengthens the thigh muscles and can improve stability. If the exercise becomes too easy, ankle weights should be added.

Isometric Ankle Exercises. Isometric exercises involve contracting a muscle without movement. An exercise band is secured to the bottom of a door and wrapped around the patient's upper foot. The patient then contracts the muscles that lift the forefoot up while sitting on the floor.

Swimming Pool Exercises. Exercising in a pool provides support for the body, allowing for an aerobic workout without the risk of falling. Walking in water also helps to strengthen the muscles used in a normal gait.

Physical therapy for foot drop is an ongoing process. The patient's physical therapist will provide a progression of exercises to stimulate increased strength and function.

Outlook for a Person with Foot drop varies

The outlook for a person with foot drop varies. The long-term development depends on the underlying cause and how long the person has had foot drop before getting treatment. In some cases, foot drop is permanent.

The outcome of physical therapy often depends on the speed with which treatment began. The person's dedication to performing exercises at home is also a major factor. With the right program, physical therapy can sometimes achieve excellent results.

Newer treatments such as FES have helped many people with foot drop to improve their gait. Surgery can also be an effective treatment in some cases, especially if a compressed nerve is causing the problem. For permanent foot drop, surgery to fuse the ankle can be useful to provide extra stability.

Foot drop doesn't always get worse with age, although there are situations where this is the case. The progression of foot drop ultimately depends on the underlying cause and treatment.

Creating a Safe Home Environment Summary

Upon returning home from the hospital and rehabilitation stay, it is imperative that the house be set up for success. Most falls happen in the home, because of environmental hazards and unsafe mobility. By creating a safe home environment, an individual will have decreased risk of falling. Starting with the entranceway to the home, a ramp may be needed to be built over stairs. If a wheelchair is needed even temporarily, doors may need to be widened or at least remove the molding. The bathrooms should be accessible for wheelchair which also would mean a wide enough door and counters that are easily reachable for care.

The home should be well lit, and nightlights should be placed in dark rooms and hallways. The local hardware store or even department stores online provide low cost motion detector lights. If getting up in the middle of the night, balance can be shaky when extremely tired and walking in the dark. When living with hemiparesis dark halls can be startling and anything unexpected on the floor can create sudden dangerous movements. Ensure that carpets and rugs lie flat. Avoid throw rugs, as these pose a significant tripping hazard. Keep floors clear and free of clutter. Cords and toys need to be kept clear. Avoid furniture with wheels and use chairs that have arm supports.

In the kitchen, frequently used items should be stored in easy to reach locations. If judgement and cognition are impaired, the stove should be removed or disabled. In the bathroom, consider a shower bench and hand-held showerhead, as well as grab bars. Place anti-skid adhesive strips to the bottom of the bathtub to avoid slipping. Long handled brushes make reaching the back much easier. Electric toothbrushes and electric razors allow for greater success with self-care and decreased risk of injury. A raised toilet seat allows for easier transfers on and off the toilet.

Behavioral and Emotional Consequences

Onset of hemiparesis and is not something anyone can truly imagine. It is not until someone acquires the loss of movement that he can truly understand how frustrating, debilitating and life changing it can be. It is normal for the individual to experience feelings of anger, loss, frustration, worrying, and sadness. Depending on the extent of disability, emotional implications can be varying. Some individuals find hope because they survived the stroke or other brain injury. Others feel anger and resentment that something so terrible happened to them. Whatever the emotion, it is important to recognize that it is normal and expected.

It is essential that the emotions are monitored and properly treated if necessary. Most people take long term antidepressant medications after onset of hemiparesis. It is also recommended that individuals seek counsel from a psychologist or counselor. This provides a healthy means of discussion and allows the individual to share his frustrations and seek guidance from a professional. Untreated depression can lead to suicidal thoughts or actions.

Impact on Caregivers and Loved Ones, Relationship Changes

When someone experiences a sudden change in their independence and physical presentation, it affects most of the people in their lives. Husbands, wives, children, parents and friends all feel a sense of loss and grieving. They usually find hope because of survival, but also mental anguish and worry as to how their lives will be changed. It is normal to worry how to care for the individual and how they will be able to financially support all the needs.

It is important to remember that there is support in the community and healthcare field, as many individuals have successfully cared for disabled loved ones. Also, it is important to study, read, and question all forms of care, therapies, and financial assistance. Utilization of public funding and disability research groups can ease some of the financial strain on families.

Loved ones may become caregivers. This can be a difficult transition for the entire family, as a wife changes her role from a partner, to a caregiver. Instead of doing things around the house together, sometimes everything is placed on one spouse. In addition, the spouse may need to assist with personal hygiene and toileting tasks, which can place embarrassment on both parties.

Relationships may change, but it is important to remember that just because of a physical disability, the individual is still the same person. It can be difficult of the individual loses memory or has difficulty recalling events and names. Provide gentle guidance and assistance and always show love. When a loved one becomes upset and loses self-esteem, it is important to reassure them of their successes and give them something to look forward to.

The best thing a loved one can do is to provide support, understanding and patience to a loved one with recent onset of hemiparesis. Let the individual be autonomous in as much as safely possible, and then give assistance. Do not try to do everything for them. This will diminish their quality of life and turn a loving relationship into that of a parent and child. Ask what the individual needs and do your best to support their needs.

Long-Term Outlook for Survivors

Unfortunately, statistics show that 40% of stroke survivors suffer serious falls within one year after stroke. Falls can lead to further brain injury, fractures, hospitalization and long-term disability. Therefore, it is essential to pay attention to safe movement and set up the living environment in a safe manner.

Practicing a safe and active lifestyle improves quality of life and overall health for stroke survivors. Participating in exercise, including strengthening and balance activities keeps the body strong to support mobility. Wearing flat, supportive shoes reduces risk of tripping. Eating a proper diet rich in calcium and protein supports bone and muscle strength. Following instructions and recommendations from the therapists ensures safety at home and in the community. Individuals should not try to walk without assistive devices or braces, as this poses significant risk for falls.

Certain medications cause unwanted side effects of dizziness, which increases fall risk. Pay attention to drowsiness and dizziness and avoid any walking if those symptoms persist.

Regular exercise helps to maintain a healthy body weight. For individuals with hemiparesis, mobility is challenging enough. If people are overweight, it causes excess strain on the joints and requires even more muscle strength to move or walk. Maintaining a healthy weight improves success with mobility. In addition, if a caregiver is needed for mobility and transfers, a healthy weight reduces likelihood of injury to the caregiver.

Research shows that during the acute stroke phase (first couple weeks), 70-80% of patients have problems with mobility in ambulation. Fortunately, at 6 months to 1 year after stroke, only 20% of patients need help from another person to walk independently. Basic activities of daily living (feeding, dressing, toileting) are compromised in 67-88% of patients in the acute stroke phase. At 1 year post stroke, only 31% of stroke survivors need another person's assistance with daily tasks.

In a study performed six months after stroke for people 65 years and older, they found that:

- 30% needed assistance for walking
- 26% needed help with daily activities of cooking, feeding, self-care
- 19% had trouble communicating
- 35% had feelings of depression
- 50% had some degree of hemiparesis
- 26% lived permanently in a nursing home

Helpful resources

Fortunately, there are many resources for individuals living with hemiparesis as well as their families. In the era of the internet, you can be overwhelmed with information, as well as support.

- HemiHelp is a website intended to provide support for children and young people living with hemiplegia and hemiparesis. http://www.hemihelp.org.uk/
- National Stroke Association is an organization dedicated to education, research, and support for individuals and families affected by stroke. http://www.stroke.org
- Children's Hemiplegia and Stroke Association is a group dedicated to young people affected by hemiplegia and stroke. http://chasa.org/
- Inspire.com is a website that shares medical conditions, support, and information as well as patient successes. This interactive website connects individuals with other people experiencing similar conditions and situations. http://www.inspire.com
- Local park districts, hospitals, community events: many park districts, libraries and hospitals host discussion and support groups for individuals affected by hemiparesis and their families.

- HELPFUL RESOURCES FORUMS SUPPORT GROUPS WEBSITES FACEBOOK GROUP TWITTER PAGES BLOGS OF INJURED, GUIDES AND BOOKS
    - Please visit http://hemiparesisliving.com/helpful-resources/

Resources are updated and added as recommended

Looking Forward with Positivity and Hope

After onset of hemiparesis, it is imperative to keep a positive outlook and be motivated to continue living life to the fullest. There are many well-known celebrities and politicians that have continued to display success after onset of hemiparesis. Some of these individuals include:

- Woodrow Wilson: The 28th president of the United States. Suffered a stroke.
- Franklin D. Roosevelt: The 32nd president of the United States. Polio left him paralyzed.
- John McCain: Due to injuries because of being prisoner of war, he has limited use of his arm and a noticeable walking impairment. He successfully served in the U.S. government and was even in a race for presidency.
- Gregg Abbott: Mr. Abbot suffered a traumatic injury when a tree fell on his back. He suffered with paraplegia of his legs. He served as a politician, governor of Texas.
- Christy Brown: An Irish author and poet. He was born with cerebral palsy that affected his motor control and speech.
- Abbey Curran: Beauty pageant winner. She was Miss Iowa 2008. Abbey was born with cerebral palsy and has motor control deficits.

A positive outlook will add significant impact to quality of life and long-term health. People with optimistic outlooks are known to life longer, healthier lives. It is important to engage with others and participate in social events. Research has shown that people who engage socially and maintain connections with support systems live a happier life with decreased episodes of depression.

Individuals should also challenge their minds and critical thinking. This can be done by learning a new skill such as music, language or an art. Reading often facilitates neuronal connections and keeps problem solving sharp. Regular exercise through strengthening, balance activities and flexibility exercises improves blood circulation, mood, sleep, and facilitates weight management. Regular exercise builds and maintains independence.

Individuals living with hemiparesis and their families should fine the good in each day, and hope for the future.

Spasticity Condition, Care, Rehabilitation Exercises and Safety

What Is Spasticity?

Spasticity is a muscle control disorder. The condition causes the muscles to become tight or stiff. Many sufferers also have lost the ability to control their muscles. In some cases, those who are suffering from spasticity may also have "hyperactive reflexes", which simply means that the reflexes are too strong. Others may have reflexes that last for too long. This condition can cause issues with normal movement, speech, and gait. It can cause pain, tightness, problems with the lower back and so much more.

While there are certainly common elements between those who have this condition, there are many variables and differences between patients.

What Are the Possible Causes?

The issue occurs because there is an imbalance in the signals that are coming from the central nervous system and that go out to the muscles. Spasticity can occur for many distinct reasons including injuries to the spinal cord, brain damage due to the lack of oxygen, stroke, encephalitis, meningitis, and traumatic brain injury. Both cerebral palsy and multiple sclerosis can cause spasticity as well.

After a Traumatic Brain Injury

After having a traumatic brain injury and damage to the brain stem, cerebellum, or the mid-brain region, there is the possibility of the development of spastic hypertonia. This can affect the reflex center of the brain and cause changes in muscle tone, reflex, sensation, and movement. The area of the brain injured will cause different areas of the body to be affected.

These types of injuries tend to be complex, and it can be difficult to treat those who suffer from spasticity that stems from TBI. The body posture could become very rigid, and one of the most common positions is to have the elbows held tightly to the sides, with the wrists and fingers bent and the fists clenched. Other times, the symptoms of spasticity that occur after a brain injury will slowly start to disappear.

Multiple Sclerosis

Spasticity is quite common with MS. There are two different types of spasticity related to multiple sclerosis - flexor and extensor. Flexor spasticity causes the knees and hips to bend involuntarily. They move up toward the chest. Extensor spasticity causes involuntary straightening of the legs. While spasticity can occur in other parts of the body, such as the arms, those forms are rarer when it comes to people who are suffering from MS.

Cerebral Palsy

People who have cerebral palsy often have damage to areas of the brain that control the muscle tone, as well as the movement of the arms and the legs. The muscles are too tense or spastic in many who have cerebral palsy. Spasticity of the muscles can cause deformities in patients as they age because they do not get as much stretching and usage as they need to through daily activities.

Stroke

Many people who have strokes find that they have spasticity in the aftermath. Strokes cause issues and damage to the brain and this often leads to spasticity, and many of the muscles are no longer capable of completing their full range of motion. As with other types of spasticity, if this goes untreated, it could lead to the muscle freezing permanently in an abnormal position.

Those who have strokes and suffer from spasticity will often find that one or both of their arms moves close to the chest, bending at both the wrist and the elbow. This can cause taking care of normal daily activities difficult for those who are trying to recover from their stroke.

What Are the Symptoms?

The symptoms of spasticity can vary from one individual to another. Be sure to know most of the symptoms that tend to manifest in those living with this condition.

- Hyperactive reflexes
- Increased muscle tone
- Involuntary movements

Many will have constant muscle stiffness. This will cause their movements to be imprecise, and it will make some tasks that require fine motor skills to be difficult to accomplish. Muscle spasms can cause painful and uncontrollable muscle contractions. These contractions can be fast, involuntary contractions that happen one after the other, or a single contraction that is sustained.

Those who have the condition will often have abnormal posture as well, simply because they are unable to hold themselves in the proper position because of the rigidity and contractions of their muscles.

Naturally, pain is also a huge factor for those who are dealing with this condition. The spasms and the contractions can be painful in many cases. Bone and joint deformities can occur as well. In some cases, a contracture can occur, which is a *permanent* contraction of the muscle and tendon. Sufferers often find that they are no longer able to take care of the normal activities in daily life, such as care and hygiene. They often need to have outside care and help.

Even if someone does not have all or most of the symptoms listed in this section, it doesn't mean that they are not suffering from spasticity. Always take the time to seek out professional medical advice for you or your loved one.

Spasticity can also cause many other potential issues in those who have the condition. These include urinary tract infections, fever, pressure sores from not being able to move properly, and chronic constipation.

What Are the Effects of Prolonged Spasticity?

Those who are suffering from prolonged spasticity, or who have loved ones who suffer, may find that the constant rigidity can cause bone and joint deformities over time. This is particularly true with those who have cerebral palsy and MS, for example. It can also change the way a person deals with the world.

As we touched upon in the previous section, spasticity can lead to pressure sores. These occur when a person is seated or laying in the same position for a long time. This causes pressure on certain areas of the body - typically the joints or the back of the head. Eventually, the skin will wear away and cause an open sore that often becomes infected.

People do not often equate spastic patients with pressure sores and bedsores, but they can and do occur. Caretakers need to be especially careful when it comes to pressure sores. In some cases, the infections can lead to death.

What Are the Treatments?

Some people who have spasticity may not even need to have any specialized treatment, especially if the case is relatively mild. However, it is important to make sure that you speak with a doctor about the best course to follow when it comes to treatments. Many patients will only need to do some regular stretching exercises to help with their spasticity and to help them to keep their range of movement. Regular stretching is an effective way to ensure that the muscles do not suffer from permanent softening.

Later in the book, we'll be covering each of the different main types of treatment in detail. These include oral medications, intrathecal medication, surgery, casts, electrical stimulation, and therapy.

Areas of the Body Affected

Many different areas of the body can be affected by spasticity. Typically, it is the legs, the upper arms, and the hands. The muscles and tendons of these areas tighten up and become rigid. Even those who suffer from mild cases of spasticity will find that it can make completing daily activities very difficult. Walking, picking something up, and doing anything that involves fine motor control are extremely difficult - sometimes impossible.

How do Doctors Diagnose Spasticity?

While the symptoms for spasticity may seem obvious, the condition needs to be evaluated by a professional. This is especially true when the symptoms are mild, as it could easily lead to a misdiagnosis if an expert doesn't perform the diagnosis. Doctors will need to conduct a full physical examination that includes neurological testing. Imaging tests tend to be quite helpful when it comes to determining the extent of the brain damage causing the injury.

Doctors use magnetic resonance imaging, or MRIs, to look at the brain and the spine. This will allow the doctors to notice any abnormalities that could cause the spasticity. The tests are very simple, but they do take time to complete. If a child needs to get an MRI, they may need to have a contrast agent administered, as this will help to make the abnormality easier to find.

Spasticity Statistics

More people around the world deal with spasticity than you might realize. Let's look at a breakdown of the spasticity statistics in the United States and around the world.

Number of People Affected in the World

According to the American Association of Neurological Surgeons, the condition currently affects more than 12 million people around the world. Out of all the people who suffer from cerebral palsy, an estimated 80% also have some degree of spasticity. The actual amount will vary based on the individual patient, of course. This is roughly 400,000 people in the United States alone. Estimates are also that around 80% of the people who are suffering from multiple sclerosis have some degree of spasticity as well. In the United States, this equates to around 320,000 people.

Number of People Affected in the United States

The number of people in the United States that suffer from spasticity of some type numbers in the millions, and the number keeps rising each year. Unfortunately, there is not always enough being done to help combat these problems, and there is little consensus on the best course of treatment. A big part of this has to do with the fact that spasticity can affect many different people with different degrees of debilitation. Doctors and therapists must look at each case individually and then determine the best course of treatment for that individual.

Number of People Who Are Diagnosed After a Stroke

According to a review in *Brain Injury* from 2013, approximately 30% of people who suffer a stroke will also have some degree of spasticity afterwards. This review looked at many different studies to come up with this number, and the percentage includes all levels of spasticity in various areas of the body.

In the United States, approximately 795,000 people a year suffer from a stroke. This means that an estimated 240,000 people have spasticity in the U.S. after going through a stroke annually.

Setting Realistic Goals for Treatment

In this chapter, we'll be covering the most commonly used methods of treatment when it comes to treatment for spasticity. However, it's first important to make sure you understand the need to set realistic goals. Treatment options will not make the spasticity vanish permanently, and it may take a lifetime of dedicated treatment to regain only a small amount of movement.

Still, working toward improving your spasticity or working with a loved one who is suffering can provide some improvement to their quality of life.

Treatment Options

Oral Medications

Oral medications have been popular with the treatment of spasticity for a long time, and they are generally the first course of treatment. Those who have stiffness and spasms that are interfering with their normal daily life will generally be prescribed oral medications that they can use. Often, these medications also help them to go to sleep, as spasticity can cause some to have trouble going to sleep at night.

Intrathecal Medication

This option, called ITB, will work better for some patients than others. It's been in use since 1992 for patients suffering from spasticity caused by cerebral palsy, MS, brain and spinal cord injuries, and stroke. This complicated but effective system uses a programmable pump that's been inserted into the patient surgically. It is possible to administer the drug right into the site of the area, and that means that the dosages are generally much lower when compared with oral meds.

Those who are candidates for this type of therapy are patients who have severe spasticity that other treatment methods, including oral methods, were unable to help. Patients who are interested in this type of therapy will need to make sure that they are good candidates by being screened by the doctor. The screening test includes getting a test dose of the meds injected through a puncture in the lumbar region and into the Intrathecal space.

During the test, the doctors will monitor the positive effects of the drug and make sure that there are no side effects. Those who have a good experience may be considered for ITB therapy.

Chemodenervation

This option requires specialized drugs to be injected directly into the muscles. The goal is to weaken or paralyze the spastic muscles. This type of treatment is often used as a part of a management program for those who are suffering from isolated spasticity. This type of treatment can work for those who are also undergoing ITB or oral meds, for example. Injections directly into the hands or arms can provide yet another measure of relief.

This type of treatment offers satisfactory results for the first couple of weeks, but the spasticity will return over time. The results will usually fade after around three or six months, when this will require another injection. However, the doctors will not usually inject the same muscle within three months because they want to avoid the creation of antibodies in the muscles, which would reduce the effects of the drug.

While there are some advantages to this option, it is important for patients to note the disadvantages as well. Namely, it has the potential to damage some of the nearby sensory nerves. Damage to these nerves could lead to pain - temporary or permanent. This could lead to a need to take more medications to deal with this new pain. It may also require surgery in some rare cases.

Surgical Treatments

Different types of surgical treatments may be possible as well. Some of the operations involved working directly with the bones, tendons, and muscles. Others involve neurosurgery. For some patients, surgery may be the best route for treatment of their spasticity.

The surgical treatment may include both neurosurgery as well as orthopedic surgery. However, not all patients will be good candidates for any of these types of surgeries for a host of different reasons. Some may have other medical conditions that make it more difficult, for example. Patients and their loved ones should speak with their doctors about the possibility of surgery for their spasticity.

Most of the surgeries will also require that the patient undergo physical therapy to get the most benefit out of the procedure.

Physiotherapy

This refers to various types of physical treatments, and it is a very common option for treating spasticity in children. Quality treatment has the potential to help reduce muscle tone and to maintain range of motion while improving coordination and strength. Many factors play a part in the success of this type of treatment, including motivation and a positive attitude, as well as the skills of the therapist.

Therapeutic treatment is available via different methods, including conventional rehabilitation. This includes stretching to improve range of motion and to reduce the possibility of contracture. This type of treatment is most effective when performed at least one or two times a day. Facilitation includes neuro-developmental therapy as well as physical therapy. Biofeedback techniques include monitoring muscle activity using a device that records whenever a spastic muscle contracts or relaxes.

Electrical stimulation has the potential to be effective as well. In these cases, it is possible to reeducate the muscles by "resetting" the balance between the extensor and flexor muscles. In the beginning, the effects will only last for about ten minutes. Many have found that after several months of using electrical stimulation, the effects will last far longer.

Casts, braces, and splints are another possibility for treatment that can work well for some. They help to support the muscles and align them, as well as to prevent or correct deformities. They can also help to reduce muscle tone and increase motion.

Which Treatment Is Right?

Everyone's case is different, and there is no "hard and fast rule" as to which type of therapy will work well for everyone. Instead, you need to speak with specialists about the options that they feel will work the best for your case.

Once they let you know which types of treatments will likely work best for you, make sure the doctors explain the procedures and potential side effects or problems that might occur. You need to be knowledgeable about medications and treatments before you or your loved ones go through with them.

Available Medications

A number of different types of medications are currently available to help with spasticity. The most common types of medications in use today are prescriptions medications, and they include both oral and intrathecal.

The intrathecal drugs include:

- Baclofen
- Lioresal
- Gablofen

The oral drugs include:

- Zanaflex
- Tizanidine
- Dantrolene
- Dantrium

You will want to speak with your healthcare professional to determine which of these medications might be right for you or your loved one.

Exercises to Help with Spasticity

Exercise and physical therapy remain workable and viable options for those who are dealing with spasticity. Even those who have undergone other treatments will find that the doctors will usually want them to include exercise to help them with their progress and to help stave off rigidity.

Typically, the best exercises involve gentle stretches that will help to relieve some of the tightness in the muscles affected. Various parts of the body will require different types of stretches naturally. It is always a good idea to have the movements be slow and controlled during the stretching process to reduce the chance of further injuring the actual muscle tissue. The best way to stretch is to slowly move the limb and hold it in the stretched position for about 60 seconds.

Some patients will find benefits from some very simple exercises including yoga. Deep breathing and meditation can help as well. Aqua-therapy can help to relieve some of the tension, and it removes the stress of weight from the body. This type of therapy is best done in cool water though, as warm and hot water can cause the muscles to tighten.

Slow strength training can help many patients with spasticity as well, especially stroke patients. A report in *Topics in Stroke Rehabilitation* mentioned that exercise will not increase the spasticity, and that it is good for relaxing and strengthening the muscles.

Any patient with spasticity who wants to add physical exercises and stretching to help deal with the condition should speak with a physical therapist that specializes in this field before beginning any exercises. This will ensure that they do not injure themselves, and that they are doing the exercises correctly to gain the most benefit from them.

Measurement of Spasticity

Measurement of spasticity is very important when trying to determine the response to the various treatments. The modified Ashworth scale, updated in 1987 by Bohannon and Smith, is the standard by which doctors will gauge the effectiveness of the treatments they are using for their different patients. The scale is simple to understand, but it takes a medical professional to make the determination of where the patient's progress or regression lays.

The Modified Ashworth Scale

- 0 = No Increase in Tone

- 1 = Slight increase in the tone. It causes a catch and release in the muscle with a small amount of resistance at the end of the range of motion when the limb is extending or flexing
- 1+ = A slightly greater increase in tone and a stronger catch before release throughout the remaining range of motion
- 2 = A much greater increase in the tone through most of the range of motion, although the limb moves easily
- 3 = A drastic increase in tone, where even passive movement is difficult
- 4 = The limb is rigid during both tension and flexion

There are other tests and spasticity charts as well. However, this tends to be the one that most of the doctors use when trying to gauge the level of spasticity and the subsequent response to the treatments.

The Emotional Consequences of Spasticity

Many times, those who have family or friends who suffer from spasticity only see the outside effects. This is sometimes true of the sufferers as well. They feel the pain, they see the pain, but they do not always consider the emotional consequences, which can often be just as devastating - and sometimes more so - than the physical consequences.

In fact, emotions can sometimes play a role in how well a person responds to treatment. Those who are down and depressed may not get as much out of the physical therapy sessions as someone who is able to maintain a positive outlook, for example. We will touch more on this in the last chapter.

What Is the Effect on Personal, Social, and Work Life?

First, let's consider the way that spasticity can affect a person's personal, social, and work life, as well as how this will in turn affect their emotional state. Because this condition reduces a person's mobility and motor skills, it means that they will not often be able to do the same things that they once did, at least not as easily. Something as simple as dancing, playing a game, or holding a child or grandchild is now not possible.

This can cause people to withdraw from doing the things that they once enjoyed, and it can put a huge damper on any type of social life. When it comes to work, the problems are just as evident. Many people find that they simply can't do the work that they once did. This makes them feel useless and helpless in many cases.

It is important to find things that you do enjoy and that you can still do. Find innovative ways to enjoy certain things, and above all, keep a positive mental outlook as much as you possibly can. This goes a long way toward improving your overall enjoyment out of life and those who share it with you.

What Is the Effect on Family and Friends?

Now, let's look at how this can affect family and friends from a couple of different angles. First, consider the person suffering from the condition. He or she may feel as though he is no longer the same person he once was, and this can cause him to withdraw from others, as mentioned above. Doing so pulls him away from family and friends who will generally want to be there and provide support.

It is also important to consider the point of view of the family and friends who are looking at their loved one who is now suffering from spasticity. Many people simply do not know how to react in these instances. They do not know how to treat the sufferer, and this can cause them to withdraw as well. It can also make some feel as though they need to walk on eggshells around the person and be careful of what they do or say.

While the circumstances of life might have changed quite a bit, that's no reason to pull away. Instead, it benefits both parties to learn more about the condition and the things they can do to help make it better, or at least a little more bearable. Find other ways to interact and still spend plenty of time with one another. After all, it's not about the *things* that you do together in the end. It's about spending time with one another and providing friendship and support through life.

What Effect Does It Have on Caregivers?

It is also very important to think about spasticity from the perspective of the caregivers who are taking care of their loved ones at home or in a facility. Caring for a loved one with this condition can be extremely draining both physically and emotionally. This is particularly true for those who have severe spasticity and who cannot move very much on their own. It is certainly hard to see someone in this condition. The caregiver will need to provide help with grooming and bathing in some cases, and even eating, not to mention at home physical therapy sessions.

Sometimes people burn out no matter how much they love and care for the person. They simply do not have the time and energy they need to provide all the care, and it can lead to bitterness beneath the surface, even though most would never admit to it. The patient often feels as though they are a burden too. If possible, it is an excellent idea to enlist some help from other friends and family members so that the primary caregiver does not have to do everything on his or her own.

If family members are not available to help, there is always the possibility of hiring someone from the outside to come in and help. This can be an expensive proposition, but hiring someone for just one or two days a week can provide the primary caregiver with enough time to recharge their batteries.

Even though it might sometimes seem as though you are making no progress, everyone involved - patient, family, and friends - needs to stay as upbeat as possible. It will help everyone in the end.

What Is the Long-Term Outlook?

The long-term outlook for those who are suffering from spasticity will naturally depend upon the severity of the spasticity, as well as the cause. Some patients can recover fully or almost fully after they've been in an accident that causes temporary symptoms of spasticity. Others have disorders that will cause them to live with it the rest of their life.

There are several treatment options available, as we've already covered. Doctors and other healthcare professionals are always looking for new ways to help their patients and to provide them with better care. With more research and medical advances, there is hope that there will be better methods of helping those who are suffering from the condition.

It's important to find ways to make dealing with the spasticity more bearable, and that's what we'll be covering in this chapter.

How Does Spasticity Affect Daily Life?

The effect that spasticity has on a person's daily life really depends on the severity. Those who have only mild spasticity will find that they are generally able to do many of the same things they've always done, albeit slower and without the ease that they once did them. Stroke patients with mild spasticity are generally able to do many of the things they once did, and therapy can help them to improve their abilities.

Those who have greater degrees of spasticity will have far more trouble. If the spasticity affects their lower body, it could lead to issues walking. Some patients will not be able to walk at all, which reduces their mobility and may confine them to a wheelchair. Those who have upper limb spasticity may no longer be able to write, type, or even hold objects.

How does all of this translate to the real world? It means that there are several different things that are no longer possible, including simple things such as bathing, grooming, and even dressing without help. Those who suffer will find that they need to have help for many of the "little things" in life. They might not be able to work in their former job, for example. This is common with many people who suffer from spasticity after they've had a stroke.

Tips for Living with Spasticity

Those who are living with spasticity should find the following tips to be helpful when it comes to improving their daily living. One of the most important things is to try to stay as mobile and active as possible. Do not let the spasticity slow you down any more than it has to. Engage in physical therapy for better health, as well as to help relieve some of the symptoms of spasticity.

It is also important to manage your stress, as this can cause the spasticity to worsen. Deep breathing exercises, tai chi, yoga, and meditation are all great, natural ways to reduce your stress levels. These can be an excellent idea for the caregiver and family members to engage in as well.

How to Create a Safe Home Environment

Keeping the home safe is very important for those with spasticity. Since each person's level of spasticity may be different, it is important to think about your *individual needs* when you are looking for ways to improve *your specific home environment*. Here are some basic tips that you can use to start.

- Use adaptive aids around the house to make reaching for objects easier.
- Install rails and nonslip flooring in the shower for better support.
- Use electric razors in the bathroom to make shaving easier.
- Electric toothbrushes can make it easier to brush your teeth even if you have limited mobility.
- Use plastic cups and utensils in the kitchen, so you do not have to worry about breaking them.
- Buy pre-sliced meat and produce.

- Make sure there is enough room to maneuver in the kitchen and bathroom for those who are in wheelchairs.
- Use transfer devices to get out of bed if needed.

Keeping a Positive Outlook

It is essential to keep a positive outlook, as we've mentioned several times in this guide. Learn to spin things in a positive direction, and try to surround yourself with other positive people. Even though you are suffering from this condition, you can't let it take away all your happiness.

Something that you may want to consider doing is joining a support group in your area. You can meet with others face-to-face or online to share your experiences and to provide encouragement for one another. Having other people to talk with who know what it is really like to live with the condition can be a huge benefit.

Resources –Spasticity Related:

http://www.webmd.com/pain-management/pain-management-spasticity

http://www.nationalmssociety.org/Symptoms-Diagnosis/MS-Symptoms/Spasticity

http://www.aans.org/Patient%20Information/Conditions%20and%20Treatments/Spasticity.aspx

http://www.medtronic.com/patients/severe-spasticity/about/

https://books.google.com/books?id=y6yCH_J5UjAC&pg=PA56&lpg=PA56&dq=What+Are+the+Effects+of+Prolonged+Spasticity?&source=bl&ots=DRALZYwhCN&sig=iWhndJyAolTeKaNQ22UOZsvjnSU&hl=en&sa=X&ei=mSSSVYynK4epNsXtgtAB&ved=0CCMQ6AEwADgK#v=onepage&q=What%20Are%20the%20Effects%20of%20Prolonged%20Spasticity%3F&f=false

http://www.medtronicneuro.com.au/movement_disorder_spasticity.html

http://cirrie.buffalo.edu/encyclopedia/en/article/32/

http://www.livestrong.com/article/488588-spasticity-exercise/

Articles and Insights from the Author's Personal Experience

Tips for Living with Hemiparesis and Avoiding Falls and Injuries

Hemiparesis Living is difficult even when you have close family support or caretaker close by. However, as we who have been injured in some way, or previously experienced **head injury or stroke, brain damage** resulting in hemiparesis, as we age, or children grow up, spouses may move apart find ourselves living alone. The detrimental effects of **hemiparesis** do not go away and with aging even exhibit stronger effects where the need for safety and extra care by one self is increased. Myself. I was shot in the head in my early twenties followed by a coma and much rehabilitation in trauma unit and hospital. I was fortunate to be able to study engineering earning my degree, but most of the two decades that followed have had me dealing with implications of living with hemiparesis and to be honest as an engineer, found myself analyzing issues that came about and finding or developing best practices or methods. I hope these insights can be used or adapted to help others going through life after head injury or **hemiparesis**.

Safety Risks and Minimizing

Starting with safety. in general, I can tell you that for myself and many spoken with in person or in online groups too, the worse effects that occur are when the body is tired. A close second is in the cold, freezing temperatures and inclement weather as snow sleet, etc.

By tired I say early in morning or especially late in the day. Arising in the night for whatever reason, can find legs extra wobbly and rather easy to lose one's balance. Having halls where light can go on easily, possibly a motion detector switch and uncluttered walkways are a couple basics that can help prevent a sudden slip or poor footing. This can really prevent serious further injury. Trust me, one shoe or slipper on a dark walkway can turn out to be a violent fall. It doesn't necessarily have to be a poor balance issue. Sometimes the weaker foot from say for example left hemiparesis or right hemiparesis will turn sideways and instead of landing on flat bottom part of foot., will land on the side of foot even at an angle sometimes. This can cause a quick fall and when this happens, a first reaction is to use the strong hand to grab onto something to catch balance. If there isn't anything on the strong side, then a fall is likely or partial fall. Keep this in mind when keeping the hall and bath safe. Railings are great, but easy to grab handles, even small ledges can help give a person's balance back. They have suction cup handles, lights that can be added economically for safety. Check a local large hardware store as Lowes.

Besides having something available on good side, simply walking slower, smaller steps will help. Walking in socks alone on some surfaces can be like walking on ice to a person with hemiparesis. For example. I can walk OK on most carpets that are wall to wall but when I approach tile or ceramic flooring or a throw rug, slow way down for safety. A common issue in people with either **left hemiparesis** or **right hemiparesis** is tripping forward when their weaker toe drags and often is close enough to floor to catch it on a carpet or even have the toes roll over. Not having proper control of these toes will look to others as not picking up the foot enough. This effect can happen so fast and somewhat unpredictable. However, going back to the first premise, this will occur more often when the body is tired or weakened in some way possibly even from extreme weather changes. It is obviously more of a possibility when walking faster. Walking faster increases the risk. Note that there are items available in stores or online to adhere throw rugs to the floors surface. This simple action can be a life saver.

Regarding Assistive Devices

Some therapists and caretakers recommend canes either a quad cane or straight cane but I can tell you after a few decades with hemiparesis, canes do not always work, they can actually give you a false sense of security causing people to move faster but not able to protect oneself in an accident. Most of the time almost always it's the weak side that has the foot dragging or catching on something, maybe a rug or object or just twisting so that it lands on the side. And what happens next is either I would fall straight ahead and to the left very fast or tip sideways again to the left. I am using left here as the weaker side or **left hemiparesis**. Now the cane would be in the stronger hand, on the right side in this case and is not much help on the left. The left arm in many of left hemiparesis won't do much good either as it is too weak to prevent the fall and probably too slow to do anything in time

If a walker is recommended and one can be modified to use with one weakened side, then use it. Of course, you'll want to learn to walk without it but for some it's best to keep using. Check with your own health professional.

In the early days after a head injury or accident, wheelchairs are commonly use and effectively safe. Myself, I've used one after the coma for almost two years before graduating to a quad cane and then later using just the regular cane and now years later without the cane during the warmer months.

<u>This last point is important with regards to wheel chairs</u>. I had lived in the snow belt up in the Northeast when I was first injured and the use of the wheelchair was indeed a life saver with the snow and ice. It is not feasible for most to leave their home areas but if possible as people with hemiparesis age, a move to the southern climate or even out west is well advised.

Living with hemiparesis and living alone can be safer in the warmer climates, free of ice and snow. That may be obvious for walking but there are other benefits as well. The sunshine daily may even help your thinking and overall attitude positively, Sure you may still get a month or two of weather where it reaches freezing but it does not stay there for long. Aches and Pains can virtually disappear. People's old injuries are often painful in cold moist weather. This is not different for head injuries, but in this case, it may very be the brain that suffers pain. It is also the control center for emotions and that too can be better in the warmer climate. **Lessons learned**.

Shower Safety After a Stroke or TBI When Living with Hemiparesis

When up to severe muscle weakness or even partial paralysis occurs on one side of the body after a stroke or traumatic brain injury, personal care cleaning oneself in a shower or bathtub is an important daily concern where steps taken before hand, during and after a bath or shower can significantly minimize any risk or unsafe practices. I cannot emphasize the importance of it enough Shower safety is reviewed with referred to facts and personal recommendations from the author, successfully living with hemiparesis for more than 30 years. The author's experience with hemiparesis living has proven that there are both inexpensive safety precautions and free advice that is invaluable when considering bath and shower safety.

Briefly, some background. Hemiparesis can be caused in several ways as most causes of hemiparesis are due to injury to the brain, from loss of oxygen. While the main cause of hemiparesis is due to a stroke, in which there is a loss of blood to a part of the brain. Other causes of hemiparesis include: trauma/falls, tumors, traumatic brain injuries, congenital defects, or birth injuries.

Safest and Most Popular Reasoning

Those affected most often are strongly independent and really need to be, especially if living alone or spending time on personal hygiene without relying on family members to help with care. An important point is that many of us do not have family living with us that can assist, and in addition it should be strongly noted that help is not always wanted, only reluctantly being asked for. Sometimes, the need for independent living overlooks proper safety, but independence and safety should be considered equally.

Seeing this, a walk-in shower is a safer option compared to baths or showers in a bathtub where one must step over the side of the tub. With a weakened side, it can be terribly awkward to enter and especially leave what can be a slippery surface. The shower is also easier for your family to assist you in or out while possibly having to lift you out of a tub.

Preparing the Bathroom for Safely Showering or Bathing

Preparation is the first step and before entering the shower an area of concern is the floor and preventing any slips or falls., Many bathroom floors are made of a tile, ceramic or polished wood and can be super slick especially for person with a weakened foot or drop foot condition. Normally for a person with drop foot or a weakened side due to injury or stroke will not have any throw rugs throughout the house. However, because of the material of bathroom floors as mentioned it is safer to cover the floor first with a carpet that would be wall-to-wall if possible. The next choice of a rug would be one with a rubber backing and affixed to the floor using some double-sided adhesion rubber or tape available at a local hardware store. Another choice would be standard bath mats with rubber backing.

Important Notes Regarding Grab Bars

In setting up the shower itself, the first consideration as certainly recommended by your own therapist would be grab bars either permanently installed with screws or the suction cup grab bar that are available in local hardware stores or your medical supply store. Of course, in your own home the permanently affixed grab bars screwed into the tile or wall are preferred and are safer. I've used these plastic grab bars myself in apartments I lived in and currently use them also.

The long horizontal bar on the shower wall is first recommended by many, however is advised here to also have a shorter bar where you enter or exit the shower or bath area. For the shorter bars, located on the shower wall entering or exiting often the plastic suction cup grab bars make sense. In the case of the suction cup adhering grab bar, I strongly recommend a redundant system though, as these are economical enough to have multiple grab bars within the shower.

In addition, it is wise to lightly tap the bars before entering a shower to double check that they are still secure. There is a caution on manufacturer boxes for these plastic grab bars to do so and from experience justly so as they will loosen up on you eventually. Be careful.

The shower or bath mat is another primary concern. It should be large, even oversize that has a gripper. If the drain hole is in the center of the shower, make sure the mat allows water to run right through it. If not water permeable when having a center drain hole in a shower, water collects on the surface, mat can become soggy and bunch up under feet. Myself, I've experienced my foot in this unsafe condition and am thankful for the grab bars when this occurred.

Hand held showerheads should be installed is this will allow one to easily reach to wash their back, under the arms or private areas.

Additional Points on Shower safety

<u>Many individuals do not have the strength or balance to take a shower standing upright,</u> For bathing. **Shower chairs and shower benches** create a safer environment for personal hygiene. The individual sits on the shower bench and uses a hand-held showerhead for washing.

<u>For individuals who can safely stand as advised by their health professional</u>

During the Shower, it is so important not to make any quick moves and always assure that your strongest foot is firmly planted on the bath mat. Your own health professional or occupational therapist would be the primary person to consult on what you should do or should not do in the shower. The author is not a medical professional but rather an engineer that has lived in a hemiparesis condition for over 30 years. The following steps may seem absurdly simple and obvious, however for a person with hemiparesis the attention to this detail can be lifesaving.

In general, sure some people use soap on a rope or a soap mit, glove to avoid soap from dropping. Others can use a liquid soap dispenser that also can be affixed to the wall with suction cups for easy one hand dispensing. However even with these options available, the soap may be dropped and probably will slip out of one's hands. The first obvious observation is to have multiple bars of soap available at hand level in the shower. It is never safe to bend over in the shower unless your strong hand is holding a secured grab bar.

After some years and gaining significant strength even in the weaker side bending over and picking something up from the shower floor can be possible safely when you follow some detailed steps. In this case, again it's advised not to make any quick movements but rather use the stronger arm to secure oneself using a grab bar or permanently affixed handle. While holding the grab bar position both feet so that the soap is in front and the soap is within a short distance possibly 6– 8 inches away. After reaching this point bend over slowly while holding a secure grab bar that is as low to the ground as possible. A quick note is that this is a good reason why multiple grab bars will allow for a safer shower. Now once you reach out and grab the soap or shampoo bottle place it on a shelf without having to stand up. This is important not to make multiple movements when you're in the shower on a weekend leg that may possibly experience drop foot. After placing the object on the shelf or ledge, with the stronger and hold on to the secured grab bar and then and only then stand up to an erect position.

Exiting the shower is dangerous especially in these cases when you land on the weekend or foot drop affected side. At some point the better leg is lifted off the ground exiting leaving the affected foot bearing the weight plus the good hand grasping the grab bar. Since the dropfoot when bare has no or little friction or grab to the floor, the location of entering and exiting should have a short 8-12-inch grab bar affixed to the shower wall or even two grab bars and positioned preferably vertically. Again, I recommend two if you are using the suction cups so that you have a redundant system that is safer.

General shower tips

Double check the water temperature with your better hand before entering the shower. During the shower wash your hair with your strong hand and if you have some grasp in your weaker hand, hold onto the grab bar with that. If the weaker hand does not have strong enough grasp, keep your feet on the bathmat and lean up against the shower wall to keep stable while washing your hair with your good unaffected hand.

After your shower, make sure your feet are firmly planted on a dry surface, rug preferably and using an oversized towel works well to dry off after a shower. A beach towel or even two smaller tiles sewed together will suffice. Another tip would be while drying off stand in front of the bed or a secured bench to avoid falling backward. This is pointed out as balance during drying movements can be unstable.

Head Injury Symptoms and Facts Victim's Families Need to Know

Head injury symptoms result from a wide range of traumatic physical conditions that affect the skull, brain, scalp and associated tissues and blood vessels. Some of these conditions are relatively mild and pose little or no threat to long-term health and wellbeing, while others pose grave threats to everyday life and normal brain function. Head injuries that impact brain health are also known as traumatic brain injuries, or TBIs. The mildest form of TBI, called a concussion, occurs when a direct impact to the head or violent shaking of the head or torso jars the brain from its normal position inside your skull. Skull fractures are TBIs that damage the heavy bones that surround and protect your brain; they can trigger bleeding or laceration of brain tissue, as well as formation of areas of bruising and swelling called contusions.

Potential Symptoms

Regardless of its cause, an injury to your head can produce relatively mild or serious head injury symptoms, according to the Ohio State University Medical Center. Common symptoms of milder injuries include bumps, bruises, small scalp cuts or lacerations, confusion, headaches, irritability, nausea, blurred vision, difficulties with body balance, fatigue, light headedness, noise or light sensitivity, lack of concentration, memory disturbances, sleep disturbances, alterations in your normal sense of taste and ringing in your ears.

Common symptoms of more severe forms of head injury include deep scalp lacerations, open head wounds, the presence of foreign objects that penetrate the scalp or skull, slurred speech, loss of consciousness, seizures, severe and persistent headaches, pale skin, walking difficulties, short-term memory loss and drainage of clear fluids or blood from the mouth or nose. Additional potential symptoms of a severe head injury include weakness on one side of the body (hemiparesis), abnormal widening or dilation of the pupil in one eye and moodiness, irritability or other changes in normal behavior.

It is important to note that not all people with head injuries develop the same types of symptoms. In addition, people who experience severe head injuries may have both mild and severe injury symptoms. For these reasons, anyone who shows any symptoms in the aftermath of a head injury should see a doctor as soon as possible. People with clear severe symptoms should receive medical care immediately.

Injury Diagnosis

In some cases, the effects of brain trauma don't show up right away. For this reason, if you have a head injury, your doctor won't necessarily be able to determine the extent of the damage without gathering several key pieces of information. Typically, she will begin collecting this information with a physical examination, complete medical history and investigation of the specific circumstances in which the injury occurred. Your doctor will also probably administer a test called a Glasgow Coma Scale, which measures your ability to open your eyes, move your arms and legs, and respond to questions and verbal prompts. The maximum possible score on the test is 15. People who score between 13 and 15 usually have only mild head injuries. People who score between 9 and 12 have moderate injuries, while those who score 8 or below have severe injuries.

Additional testing procedures used in a TBI diagnosis include blood tests, X-rays, a measurement of the brain's electrical activity called an electroencephalogram (EEG), a combination of X-rays and computer imagery called a computed tomography (CT) scan, and a magnetic resonance imaging (MRI) scan, which uses radio frequencies, computers and specialized magnets to generate detailed pictures of the brain.

Changes in Consciousness

The presence of a brain injury can alter your normal consciousness in several different ways. Some people develop a temporary reduction of conscious responsiveness called lethargy or stupor, which can typically be overcome with some sort of strong body manipulation or stimulation. A more serious form of consciousness alteration - called a coma - stems from widespread, scattered forms of brain damage and results in loss of awareness and a lack of responsiveness to all outside stimuli. Some people in comas recover consciousness in days or weeks, while others die or enter another state of consciousness called a vegetative state.

Unlike people in comas, people in vegetative states sometimes open their eyes, experience periods of relative alertness, move their bodies and respond reflexively to outside stimulation. In many cases, vegetative individuals regain some conscious function in several weeks. However, in other cases, vegetative patients show no signs of change for 30 days or longer, and therefore enter another state of consciousness alteration known as a persistent vegetative state. Adults who enter this state have roughly a 50 percent chance of improving and regaining consciousness in the next six months, while children have roughly a 60 percent chance of recovering. If a persistent vegetative state lasts for more than a year, the affected individual has very little chance of regaining consciousness. Those who do regain consciousness after this amount of time typically have significant or severe disabilities and require ongoing rehabilitation in order to gain even small improvements in everyday function.

Trauma Head Injury: Symptoms and Recovery Process

Trauma head injury occurs when the head is subject to a blow or a wound. When a person suffers a trauma head injury, it should be assumed that the brain is also affected. Because of this, it's imperative that any traumatic head injury be evaluated by a medical professional as soon as possible.

Symptoms

The symptoms of traumatic head injury can vary. If the injury is mild, the patient might experience unconsciousness that lasts no more than a few minutes. Some people don't lose consciousness but are just disoriented or a bit dazed. The patient might have a headache, might have trouble concentrating and lose some of their memory. They might be nauseated, be sensitive to light, be depressed, anxious or moody. They might be drowsy or suffer from insomnia or clumsiness.

People who suffer from more serious traumatic head injuries can be unconscious for several hours. They might not even be able to be awakened. When awake, they might have very dramatic behavioral changes. They might be very confused, have severe and unceasing headaches as well as nausea and vomiting that won't stop. They might suffer from seizures. One or both pupils may be "blown" or dilated, and they might have clear fluid leaking from their ears or their nose.

Children's symptoms may be different as very young children don't have the language to describe their symptoms. Babies might not nurse the way they used to. They may cry incessantly and be irritable. Their sleep habits might be altered. Older children might seem to be depressed and have no interest in things that gave them pleasure before. They might not be able to pay attention as well as they used to.

Recovery Process

After the patient has been treated for the initial injury, he or she may need to undergo a recovery process. With a mild injury, all the patient may need to do is rest for a few days and take pain meds to treat any headaches. Still, even a patient with a mild injury needs to be watched to make sure his or her symptoms don't worsen. The doctor will let the patient know when he or she can return to normal activities.

Other patients who have more severe injuries might need rehabilitation. This starts even before the patient is released from the hospital and continues in inpatient or outpatient rehabilitation services. The professionals that may be called upon to help the patient include:

• A pathologist who specializes in speech and language and is there to help the patient recover his or her communication skills.

• An occupational therapist who helps the patient relearn day to day tasks.

• A physical therapist who helps the patient to walk again and regain his or her balance if it's been lost.

• A psychiatrist or a neuropsychologist who supports the patients behavioral, psychological and emotional skills.

• A vocational counselor who tries to help the patient return to work or to find job opportunities.

• A physiatrist, who's a physician who oversees the patient's recovery and rehabilitation. He or she might work with a nurse who specializes in trauma head injury. This nurse also works with the patient's family and is a liaison between members of the patient's support team.

Receive FREE a Special Report for Head Injured and Caretakers which Reveals MUST KNOW patient and caregiver resources, potential symptoms, behavioral and emotional consequences, steps in rehabilitation, creating a beneficial home environment, brain injury medications, long-term outlook, and more, http://www.hemiparesisliving.com

Author Leon Edward at his Website presents checklists for people with head Injury, hemiparesis and Stroke plus tips, articles from well-known professionals and authors in the field plus blogs on his own experiences with over two decades living and working with head injured, hemiparesis and stroke effected.

Head Injury and Employment Workplace Communication from a TBI Survivor

Fortunately for people with a head injury of various degrees, today there are more opportunities for employment. However, there still are issues that are both visible and many that are internal to the people with the head injury. Communication in the workplace is often one of the most valued skills among professionals while mis-communication can be damaging in customer relations especially, costly in some projects or detrimental for interpersonal communication among coworkers.

<u>Common Symptoms Effecting Spoken Communication that Vary in Degree</u>

Communication afterward can be affected in various degrees after mild to severe head injuries, some may be visibly or audibly obvious as in speaking clearly or possibly slowly, sometimes extremely slowly. More common are problems in auditory processing, memory, people skills, fatigue at times, mood swings and focusing one's attention as concentration. Focus and concentration are key here in contributing to communication of head injured as I have been. There are even times when words or phrases may be spoken out of order and can be awkward when spoken. Also controlling various emotions can sometime be an issue in employment as well if not evident to others, well certainly internally.

All these have occurred to me at various times, with improvement in some areas after much exercise, self-help audios or even talk with loved ones or therapy with professionals. Other areas are an ongoing issue yet minimized through techniques, exercises, sometimes strategies for almost three decades now with tips listed in article.

Sure, people react and live their lives differently but head injured do have common physical and especially mental effects that are exhibited similarly but to different degrees. Also, it is interesting how people in different professions, ages, in different work environments really act differently towards a person exhibiting one or more of the detrimental effects listed previously.

<u>Slow Speech at times and Communication in the Workplace</u>

At times, the thought processing and speech can be slow. but not constantly slow. It could be termed inconsistent speech and draw attention to an issue in this way. During verbal communication on the job or even during employment interviews, talking one speed and then suddenly slowing down drastically may call attention to the issue especially if the other person is unaware of any past physical injury, the head injured person can look as if they are ignorant of the topic when it just doesn't always come out or is spoken as fast and as clear as it should be. Even when coworkers, managers or customers have known of my TBI from years ago, they can act unacceptably. The most common reaction amongst people who work with me is to finish my sentences for me or restating it as "this is what he meant". They may be trying to be helpful but sometimes make me angry on the inside or wanting to say that their version is not what I meant. But more than likely time is limited and talking slow or hesitating for the right words just has no place in some high paced work environments.

I can tell you that this can be an extremely frustrating event when knowing the answer or correct response that may be beneficial to a conversation yet not being able to verbalize it fast enough. Some others will just talk right over you while a few will give time for the injured to answer. Frustration can even turn to anger on the inside more quickly for some depending on their own injury. I know this has occurred for me and keeping calm is something that was not easy when I was younger. The point of bringing this up was that since I have minimal control of the times when I may hesitate, looking for the right word or thought, I speak in a slower speed or speech pattern most of the time. Most others will allow you to finish thoughts when you do speak slower in general. Though, there are a few who just will still cut you off before you are finished to get their own thoughts across. If possible, stating that you were not finished is often a helpful phrase to use depending on the other persons position or status in the company.

Sure, knowing what to say but not being able to verbalize it fast enough is a common cause of the slow speech intervals but the brain processing is slower in general. Hesitating for the right word to speak can be why speech is slower at times. As mentioned, by using the technique or practice of speaking slower during meetings or interviews, the moments of slower recall of words can be effectively minimized or it will not look as bad.

This is another area where smart coworkers can recognize a difficulty in processing speed or do things slower so they talk slower and talk to you or sometimes as if you are a child. When it happens to me I feel like stating that I'm no child and even though I act slow, I'm rather intelligent with an engineering degree and much technical training. I've even had a manager or colleague belittle me while talking to me in front of other managers or coworkers. Sometimes one cannot avoid other reactions but learn to handle it better. For us with the head injury, quiet meditation, gratefulness and prayer daily can help immensely.

Author Leon Edward at his website at HemiparesisLiving.com presents articles. free resources, Checklists and tips from well-known professionals and authors in the field plus blogs on his own experiences with over 30 years living and working with hemiparesis.

Acquired Brain Injury Can Result in Behavioral and Emotional Consequences

Apart from any specific behavioral or emotional difficulties, people with head injuries or acquired brain injuries typically go through many emotional changes as they adapt to their new circumstances. In the immediate aftermath of their injuries, patients commonly experience a great deal of confusion, as well as an agitation with their unfamiliar internal and external environment. The struggle to deal with such a profoundly altered situation and brain injury symptoms may cause even the most mild-tempered person to lash out physically at those nearby. In most cases, this confused state will diminish or disappear entirely within anywhere from days to months.

Brain-injured people also frequently develop an attitude of denial toward their situation. Sometimes, this denial manifests in people who have undiagnosed problems in the aftermath of an accident. At other times, it manifests in people with diagnosed cases of brain damage. While denial has a strong emotional component, it can also reflect a true inability to recognize the fact that something's wrong. For instance, some forms of brain trauma limit self-awareness and the ability to notice changes in perception. In addition, undamaged portions of the brain can contribute to this problem by following automatic routines that effectively "hide" the presence of serious malfunctions.

Usually, blanket denial eventually gives way to a mixed state of anger and depression. Bursts of anger can stem from actual physical changes inside the brain that reduce normal levels of emotional control. However, anger and depression can also stem from a recognition of changed circumstances and a feeling of helplessness about remedying those circumstances. In some cases, brain-injured people blame themselves for what's happened to them; this is especially true for those involved in risky behaviors such as drinking and driving. In other cases, people with brain injuries blame another person who caused their accident, or blame some larger, unknowable force or fate.

Behavioral problems commonly associated with acquired brain injury or more generally head injured can include violence or other forms of aggression, failure to comply with prompts or requests, diminished self-awareness, diminished self-control, inappropriate behavior, egocentric or childlike behavior and an unwillingness to take responsibility for one's actions. Common emotional problems include anger, confusion, depression, mood swings, apathy, agitation, frustration, paranoia, irritability and anxiety. In some cases, combined emotional and behavioral problems grow severe enough to warrant a diagnosis of a condition called borderline personality disorder.

People with even mild or moderate brain damage commonly experience disruptions in their normal ability to remember, think and reason. People with more severe forms of damage may have extensive problems in these areas, as well as problems expressing themselves, understanding what's being said to them and processing information from any or all the five senses. Most people who suffer traumatic brain injuries also have significant psychiatric problems that manifest as changes in their behavior or emotional state.

Some people remain permanently angry and/or depressed in the aftermath of their injuries. However, others improve through rehabilitation and start to test the limits of their returning mental and motor skills. While this testing is vital for maximizing the potential for recovery, it can also lead to its own denial or sense of frustration as patients with significant remaining problems seek to gloss over those problems and focus only on their successes. For example, a person with diminished levels of energy may decide to ignore this problem and attempt to get a lot of things done in a relatively brief period. In turn, this overexertion can result in fatigue that lingers for days and leaves the person feeling like a "failure." Unnecessary feelings of failure can also set in if a brain-injured patient has unrealistic expectations about the pace of rehabilitation and doesn't reach a self-directed goal or milestone in a certain amount of time.

In some cases, people with brain injuries eventually come to accept their limitations, brain injury symptoms and the pace of their rehabilitation. For those with temporary problems, this can mean dealing with short-term difficulties on the way to a full recovery. However, for those with permanent impairments, it means making ongoing adjustments to a new reality and learning how to regain a sense of self that will sustain them in the future. On a physical level, this type of adjustment involves working within the known capabilities of the body. On an emotional level, it can involve forging new relationships with friends, family and acquaintances, as well as forging a new internal self-image

Brain Food and Nutrients for Your Mind

Brain Food is any food that is an aid in a person's intelligence. Therefore, brain food is food that affects your intelligence, creativity, memory, or any other intellectual part of your life. Eating a diet with the right brain foods might seem like too much work, but, it is something that is easy to do. You want to be sure that as an adult you are eating great brain food, and that your children are exposed to a diet that provides them with the strong brains they need to grow and thrive.

It might not be something that you are aware of, but the food that you eat does affect the performance of your brain. It has been proven that if you are able to eat the right foods, you will be able to boost your IQ and do things like improve your mood, be more emotionally stable, and sharpen your memory, along with keeping your mind young and healthy. Therefore, eating correct foods is one natural way that you can make sure your brain is healthy, which will lead to a much healthier life for you, overall.

If you can give those correct nutrients to your brain, you will find out that you can think quicker, and can also have a better memory. Not only that, but you'll be able to be better coordinated and have better balance, as well as being able to concentrate better. These factors are extremely important for you, so be sure that you are following through and eating healthily.

There are several key brain foods that you can eat which will do these things, and boost your brainpower so that you can be healthy and happy. However, before you begin to think about the foods that you must eat for a healthy brain, you should think about the factors that influence a healthy brain. Keeping these factors in mind is the best way to make sure you are doing as much as you can to have a healthy mind. To have a healthy brain, there are three main ingredients. You need to drink lots of water, get lots of air, and eat the right foods.

Brain Factors for Health

1. Water

Water is the first part of a healthy brain, and of healthy brain foods. You need to be able to have the right allowance of water in your blood to have a healthy brain. Your brain must be fully hydrated so that it can provide you with the right-thinking skills. The circuitry in your brain relies on being well hydrated so that it can perform its functions well. Be sure that you are drinking plenty of water. You will know if you are dehydrated because you won't sweat as much, you might get a headache, and you will feel tired. Your brain feels tired as well, and can't perform its functions fully when it isn't hydrated. So, keep yourself, and your brain, in plenty of water. Eating smaller meals and snacks is a terrific way to keep the H2O in your brain where it belongs.

2. Air

Air is another thing that your brain needs to survive. Obviously, you need air to stay alive, but your brain needs more air than just enough to keep it living, to be healthy. You might not think that you knew this, but there has always been a simple clue. After you eat a big meal, the air in your body is all being concentrated to your stomach to help digest the food, and therefore you end up feeing sleepy now. The more air that you can get into your brain, the more alert and awake you are going to be in your life. Therefore, to have a healthy brain, be sure that you are getting fresh air each day and never depriving yourself of it. If you eat smaller meals, your body will not have to send as much oxygen to your stomach and your brain can stay alert and awake all day long.

3. Brain Foods

Thirdly, you want to focus on the food that you eat to keep your brain healthy. Brain foods are also important to understand because they can help you be more alert, be smarter, and even more creative. The best things that you can do for your brain include eating the right foods during your life. If you can eat well for your brain, your brain will be able to take care of you for as long as you are alive. Keep careful track of the food that you eat, and don't skimp out on the important foods.

Neurotransmitters

The neurotransmitters in your brain are what is responsible for all the functions that you hold so dear. There are neurotransmitters that oversee the way that you move, the way that you think, and the way that you feel. Each of them needs to be treated well – and fed well – so that they can provide you with the best work possible. There are three key neurotransmitters, and eating the right foods will help each of them succeed.

Acetylcholine

Acetylcholine is the first one. It is responsible for the voluntary movements that your body makes. It is also responsible for drinking, memory, and behavioral inhibitions. People who have Alzheimer's and memory loss might have less Acetylcholine, or the transmitters might be blocked. To keep your brain healthy and to keep your mind and memory sharp, you need to be sure that you are providing your brain with high Acetylcholine levels. To do this, eat lots of egg yolks, peanuts, wheat germ, meat, fish, milk, vegetables and cheese. They contain plenty of Acetylcholine.

Dopamine

The next important neurotransmitter is dopamine. It oversees your voluntary movement and emotional arousal. Schizophrenia might be associated with having too much dopamine, and having too little might be something that causes Parkinson's disease. The drug L-Dopa is given to increase the levels of dopamine in the brain.

Therefore, it is important that you do all you can to keep the levels of dopamine correct in your brain. To have elevated levels of dopamine, eat meat and milk products, as well as fish and beans, nuts and soy products. In fact, eating 3 or 4 ounces of protein will help you to be more energized, and will make you more alert and even more assertive.

Serotonin

Serotonin is involved with arousal, sleep, mood, appetite, and sensitivity. It is also something that is excitatory, and is part of how the brain produces feelings of pleasure. Depression might be caused by having too little serotonin that is active in the brain. To keep your levels right and to keep them active, eat lots of pasta, starchy vegetables, potatoes and cereals, as well as breads.

Eat for Intelligence

Aside from taking care of the neurotransmitters in your brain, there are also other things that food can do for you. There are some important tips that you can follow to be overall smarter and to eat for intelligence. First, balance your glucose levels. This means that the levels of sugars in your body must be level so that your brain can work well. Secondly, eat the fats that are essential to your diet. Third, include plenty of protein, and fourth, include plenty of vitamins. Along with this, there are some key areas to be sure that you include.

Protein

Protein is important in balancing your brain health. It provides the building blocks for your body, and for your mind. Protein is also used to make the neurotransmitters in the first place. It is found in meat, fish, milk and cheese. It provides the building blocks for the way that your body will grow and change, so it is important to all your body systems. It helps the body's tissues, internal organs, nerves, and brain and heart thrive. Eating protein will help you have improved mental performance.

Neurotransmitters

First, you must focus on the neurotransmitters that can be found in your brain. There are three key neurotransmitters, and eating the right foods will help each of them succeed.

Acetylcholine is the first one. It is responsible for memory, and movement, as well as behavioral inhibitions. To keep this healthy, eat lots of egg yolks, peanuts, wheat germ, meat, fish, milk, vegetables and cheese. They contain plenty of Acetylcholine.

The next important neurotransmitter is dopamine. It will help with your voluntary movement and emotional arousal. To have high levels of dopamine, eat meat and milk products, as well as fish and beans, nuts and soy products.

Serotonin is involved with arousal, sleep, mood, appetite, and sensitivity. To improve this in your brain, eat lots of pasta, starchy vegetables, potatoes and cereals, as well as breads.

Carbohydrates

Carbohydrates are also important to a healthy brain. They enhance the absorption of tryptophan. This is converted to serotonin, and is used in the brain. If you eat a carbohydrate meal, you will feel calm and relaxed for several hours. The key carbohydrates that you can eat are grains, fruits, and vegetables. Also, digestion causes the breakdown of carbohydrates in to the glucoses or sugars that your body needs. This is also the primary source of energy for your brain in general. If you don't keep your glucose levels even, which means your carbohydrates are out of whack, you might feel confused, dizzy, and you might also have convulsions or lack of consciousness.

Fat

Fats are also an important part of your brain health. This is because the brain itself is more than 60% fat. The reason that the brain contains so much fat is that the brain cells themselves are covered by something called the myelin sheath, which is made up of 75% fat. Fat is an important messenger in your brain, and is responsible for regulating your immune system, the way that your blood circulates, and memory and move. Omega 3 fatty acids are essential to the way that your brain performs. You can find Omega 3 fatty acids in oily fish like salmon, sardines, and tuna. You can also find it in Flax seed and in vitamin

Vitamins and Minerals

Vitamins and minerals are also important for a healthy brain. They are essential for the way that your brain grows and develops. If you truly want to have a healthy brain, you need to be able to get plenty of B vitamins. These are the vitamins that are responsible for making your brain healthy and producing energy for your entire body. A, C, and E vitamins are antioxidants, and are very important for preserving memory in the elderly, as well as in people at any age.

Important minerals that you need to promote good brain healthy include magnesium and manganese. These are important for brain energy. Also, Sodium, potassium and calcium are important as well to strengthen the thinking process. These minerals also make sure that the transmission processes that your brain does daily go off without a hitch and continue to work just as well as they can.

It is often hard to figure out the important things that your body needs at all stages to be as healthy as possible. However, if you can keep your brain hydrated, with enough air, and with the proper foods, you'll find that your brain is healthier. When your brain is healthy, so is your entire body. Therefore, brain food is never something that should be taken lightly, because it is not something you want to ignore. Remember that the correct balance of foods is important. There isn't one main food that is a brain food, or that will promote the best brain healthy. A combination of proteins, carbohydrates, fats, and vitamins and minerals is essential for good brain health. It is also important to eat the correct foods so that your neurotransmitters can function as well as possible. Even though it might seem like a brain food diet is difficult to understand or to do, it really is quite simple. And eating a diet like this will provide you with the best healthy that you can ever imagine.

.

The Importance of Rest and Sleep on Concentration

Getting enough rest and sleep is key to overall function. Studies have concluded that most people are not getting enough meaningful rest and sleep. Proper rest is necessary as during this time, the body goes into a sort of reparative state. It reboots itself so that a person can function at optimum capacity.

Most people are not getting enough rest and sleep. This can potentially cause major health issues such as lowered immune system, obesity, heart disease, etc. When a person does not get adequate amounts of proper sleep and rest, it more than just a matter of feeling tired. It can affect a person's ability to concentrate.

More scientific studies are being done to get a more accurate measure of how lack of sleep can affect concentration. It is estimated that for a person to have adequate concentration abilities, adults need 7 to 8 hours of sleep and for adolescents between the ages of 11 and 22, nine and a half hours of sleep are needed. When a person gets less than 6 hours of sleep, the ability to concentrate is significantly reduced. This lack of concentration not only affects things like being able to remember what tasks need to be performed at work or school, and remembering which items a person may need from the grocery store. Lack of rest and sleep affects a person's ability to react in potentially dangerous situations. If someone has not had adequate rest, he or she may not be able to drive a car properly. A person who operates dangerous machinery for a living may lose the ability to concentrate, thus putting not only himself or herself at risk, but also risks the safety of other employees. If your healthcare professional is functioning on inadequate amounts of sleep and rest, he may render an incorrect diagnosis which puts you at risk for receiving unnecessary testing, procedures, or medications. It also puts that medical professional at risk of losing licensure due to negligent and improper treatment of his patients. Similar concerns arise with those who are employed in the transportation industry. If an airline pilot, train conductor, or taxi driver is not fully rested, he or she and the company for which they are employed could be held liable for negligence.

Getting adequate rest and sleep is not just about feeling good, though feeling good is certainly a sign that a person is well-rested. It also has to do with being able to function and concentrate on varying tasks at optimal levels throughout the day.

There are some suggestions from health professionals on getting to sleep, getting quality sleep and even getting back to sleep in the middle of the night. Some may seem obvious but if we aren't consciously aware of these causes, effects can be damaging to your mental focus.

Helpful tasks to sleep better are keeping a regular bedtime, consuming dairy products where warm is better, reading dull material, sleeping in absolute darkness, maintaining quiet and more detail is available from other sources. Don'ts include food additives, avoiding protein and sweeteners.

Four Elements of Concentration

You'll find, when it comes to concentration, there are four elements that help to define it. These are the:

- Width
- Direction
- Intensity
- Duration

The width of your attention must do with the amount of information coming at you from all sources. That means that it can be a rather wide perspective, with a great deal of information directed at you, or simply a narrow perspective, where it's just a limited amount, trying to get your attention. Being able to grasp a lot of information at the same time takes practice, and even more so to shift from a large amount to a small amount and back again. Learning to do this however, will help you to avoid the unimportant thoughts that everyone experiences all day every day, and really hone in on what's important, to focus your thoughts.

The second component of attention is direction. This means how well you can filter information and events as they come at you. There are times when it's just not possible to filter out all events changing around you. This too requires practice.

The third component, intensity, can vary from moment to moment. Concentration can go from very weak to incredibly intense, depending on the situation in which you find yourself. Again, it requires practice to go from weak attention to detail, to an intense, focused concentration.

The last component is the duration of your attention. It can go from brief to long, sustained intervals of time. Keep in mind that it's not always possible to maintain extended periods of intense, focused attention. In fact, the more intense the attention, the shorter the duration you can maintain it.

The length of a person's attention span is on average between twenty and ninety minutes, depending of course, on the person's interest in the subject at hand.

As early as 1890, William James had already formed a definition of attention. He said, "Everyone knows what attention is. It is taking possession by the mind, in clear and vivid form, of one out of what seems several simultaneously possible objects of trains of thought: focalization, concentration of consciousness is its essence. It implies withdrawal from some things to deal effectively with others."

Since then, students, athletes, business men and women, psychologists, scientists, and researchers have used everything in their arsenals to increase their ability to focus their minds on the task at hand, whatever is relevant at that moment in time, to the exclusion of all else. Athletes, intent upon their sport, must focus their mind and body, like a laser beam on the appropriate action, pushing everything else from their minds. Only by doing so will they win the game; no time to daydream here.

In sports, as with other endeavors, the play changes by the second and athletes must be focused on what they are doing, fully aware and ready to spring into action, change course, and win the game. Nothing else is acceptable. There is no room in the sports arena for daydreamers. Athletes call this ability to hone in with laser-like ability being 'in the zone.'

Dr. Robert Nideffer, psychologist and founder of Enhanced Performance Systems has classified the two rudimentary categories of attention as internal and external. He describes internal attention as mentally projecting oneself into the proposed action, whatever problems might be encountered.

External attention is, of course, what is going on around oneself. An example would be a member of a team, being constantly aware of where his/her teammates are at any given moment, as well as those on the opposing team.

Athletes, probably better than anyone else, learn how to focus on the moment, to the exclusion of all else.

How are we able to focus on and deal with all the information coming at us at once? Research shows that we deal with this information on two levels. One is simply automatic; we grab onto it without consciously thinking about it. This generally happens when we are performing tasks that we have learned over time and can do almost by rote.

The second level we work at is called the controlled level. This is limited by the capacity of the brain to deal with all the information available to us. If we go beyond that capacity, our performance automatically declines. It is even possible to work on both levels at the same time, though of course, the automatic level works much faster than the controlled level.

The trick is to bring oneself to a state of awareness and energy, directed towards the desired goal. Some athletes or those involved in other types of contests might find themselves over-excited to the point of distraction. They experience nausea or nervousness, which naturally distracts them from their original focus.

How to Increase Concentration and Focus with Exercise

It seems that today there is a clear need for increased emphasis on the importance of exercise. Because of the realization of the importance of exercise as a path to health and wellness, the fitness industry has seen tremendous and sustained growth over the past few years. While physical fitness is incredibly important and necessary for wellness, one aspect of exercise is being unfortunately overlooked: Exercise that trains the mind. By focusing on the following exercises, one can improve their abilities to focus and concentrate, while also sharpening their recall. Listed below are the 5 best exercises how to improve concentration and focus:

Visual Exercise

For this visual exercise, the user will require two differently colored pencils and a timer equipped with an alarm. Set the timer to go off at varying intervals, so that during one interval the alarm will go off after 12 seconds, and during the next it will go off after 8 seconds, and so on. The user will hold one pencil in each hand, and extend one arm out so that the hand is at eye level, focusing upon the pencil. When the alarm goes off, the user will switch arms and focus upon the other pencil. This exercise trains the visual cortex of the brain, which helps the user focus while also ignoring any potential distractions.

Meditation

This isn't the traditional form of meditation. Instead, the user will pick out any object before beginning the meditation session, and will study the object for an extended period, maybe about 10 minutes. They will look at all angles of the object, taking mental note of every detail such as its shape, contour and color. The user will then close their eyes and attempt to visualize the object by recalling all their mental notes. This exercise helps to greatly improve memory recall and concentration.

Scent Observation

This next exercise may require the user to take a walk outside where there is plenty of plant life. On this walk, the user should pay close attention to all the scents they observe, trying to identify each one. After a brief period, they should select one of the scents they have observed and identified and try to smell only that scent. By concentrating on that single scent, the user will be able to greatly increase their ability to focus on a single thing while tuning out any potential distractions. This skill can be applied to all the senses, not just smell.

Mirror Focus

This exercise may bring to mind Robert DeNiro's character in *Taxi Driver*, but one must trust that this is a perfectly normal and healthy exercise. While looking into the mirror, one should draw circles around the reflection of the eyes. Focus should be directed into the reflection of the eyes, attempting to remain perfectly still. While maintaining this stillness, the user should focus only on breathing deeply while maintaining focused attention on the reflection of the eyes. This exercise will not only improve focus and concentration, but will also impact the user's level of confidence.

Physical Exercise

It has been demonstrated time and again that physical fitness activities dramatically improve brain function when a user engages in these activities on a consistent basis. By incorporating any type of physical fitness routine, brain functions such as concentration and focus are positively impacted. Many physical fitness activities are great opportunities for introspection or brainstorming. While engaging in certain activities such as running or cycling, many users report that the physical stimulation causes their brain to feel equally stimulated, which result in some of their best thoughts and ideas. This is backed up by scientific studies that show 10 to 40 minutes of exercise can lead to an immediate boost in concentration and focus.

If one has a desire to improve their brain function, particularly their ability to focus and concentrate, simply engaging in the above activities will make a noticeable difference. By taking just a few moments from their day, users can take joy in the fact that they are able to focus more closely and concentrate much more thoroughly than they were ever able before.

More Tips for Laser Like Focus and Concentration

When you set goals for yourself, whether it is in rehabilitation, exercises, is in school or the workforce, it is important that you concentrate on the task at hand to obtain those objectives. For millions of people, it is not that easy.

It is difficult to obtain your objectives if you do not know what they are. It is necessary to
define what your goals are. This will assist you obtaining them. When you have clear and concise objectives, you will be able to focus and concentrate better.

When you take on too many tasks at one time, you are setting yourself up for failure. Overwhelming yourself with too many tasks will inhibit your ability to focus because you will stress about getting everything done on time. Doing one thing at a time will help you to concentrate better.

If the task that you have is a big one, breaking it down in segments will assist you in completing more competently. Focus on the segment that you are working on and not the whole project. Concentrating on the task in front of you will allow you to complete it correctly with very little stress, and often, you can complete it before the deadline.

No matter who you are, expect the unexpected. There are no guarantees that you are going to have an error proof life. Obstacles always crop up and you need to be prepared to handle whatever is thrown at you to meet your goals. Distractions are all around us every day, being able to shut them out and concentrate on your task will assist you in completing it quickly and efficiently.

Success and recognition is gained over time. Nothing worth having is easy. You need to be able to concentrate and do the very best that you can in everything that you do. It is important that you do not give in to stress, it will only slow you down and concentration will be difficult if not impossible. Sometimes taking a short break will help you to regain your focus and concentration. You may find that by doing this, your focus will improve.

To be a success, sacrifice is sometimes required. It is like an exchange. You will give up one thing to gain another. You just need to make sure that what you give up is worth what you are gaining. If you have a job that requires you to focus intensely on your task, you may want to remove the telephone from your desk, as each time it rings, your concentration is broken. When you remove the daily distractions, you are doing something that can help you to focus on your job.

Putting things off is the number one cause of stress. When you put things off, they tend to creep up on you all at once and you find yourself with a multitude of tasks that need to be finished all at once. This not only causes stress that leads to loss of concentration, it also can cause you to become overwhelmed with work, and that can lead difficulties in focusing. When you do what you are supposed to do at the time you are supposed to do it, you will find that your concentration will be stronger.

Brain Gym Training to Increase Memory Capacity Concentration and Improve Thinking Even Linguistics

While many spend substantial amounts of time, money and energy on developing their physical strength, few realize that their mental capacity can be similarly developed and strengthened. We often feel like we are simply stuck with what we're given mentally, but that is not the case. While we all are born with certain innate cognitive abilities, there are many exercises you can engage in to increase your mental faculties just as you would your physical ones. Think of it as brain gym training.

People of all ages, types of employment, student or professional are optimizing their mind brain and thought power today. Here's a look at specific exercises and activities that will aid brain improvements when practiced regular and are no cost.

Memory

Memory is a pivotal component of all cognitive activities, from reading to calculation and reasoning. There are many different types of memory at work in the brain. You need to train if you want to maintain a good memory. Luckily this is not difficult as it may seem at first. Acetylcholine, a chemical that helps build the brain, is enhanced every time you memorize the lyrics to a new song. This helps increase memory capacity. Other challenges that can help include using the non-dominant hand to perform mundane activities and performing daily tasks without the aid of light.

Concentration

Focus is essential to all cognitive tasks. The ability to sustain attention amidst external distractions aids greatly in the ability of the brain to take on new mental challenges. By simply changing up your routine, you can improve attention. Simple changes such as taking a new route to work or reorganizing your workspace can wake your brain up to stay attentive. As we age it can become easier to get distracted. By combining activities such as running while listening to podcasts or doing math in your head can push your brain to maintain optimal levels of concentrative ability.

Linguistic

Language activities can train up our ability to recognize patterns in speech and remember and understand words. They also can boost your fluency, grammatical skills and vocabulary. With sustained effort, you can broaden your knowledge of new words and increase the time of retrieval for familiar ones. Change up your reading so that you are exposed to new language patterns and words. This will increase your mental flexibility and word use, making language more fun and expressible.

Stay Sharp

These are a few things you can do to immediately begin developing and strengthening your brain. Brain gym training can be just as effective as a regular exercise or training at the gym, as your mind is just as necessary a tool in your daily functioning in life as your physical capacities. Keep your mind sharp so that you will be on top of your game and ahead of your peers even in old age. You can maintain your cognitive abilities longer than your physical ones, and in the long run your mind will be your greater asset

Improving Your Memory with Brain Exercises, Brain Games

Memories can be a very basic part of us because they literally make up a large part of who we are. We remember good and tough times, memorable times, and so on Engaging in brain exercises to keep your memory sharp can help.

Among the best things you can do to improve your memory are to play memory games. For example, matching two like things with an array of cards that you have laid out facing down in front of you is one good game to play. If you turn over two of them, you get to move them away from the remaining cards. If they don't match, you turn them face down again, and then go on to the next card. The idea of this game is to remember where you've seen cards that you've turned up and then turned back down so that you can match them up with "buddies" when you turn those over. You can play this game online as well as with physical decks of cards. With the online games, simply click your mouse over the "face down" cards to turn them over, and again to turn them back to facing down.

Another great way to improve your memory is via association. With this scenario, you relate something new to something familiar. As one example, you can associate a person's name with something that reminds you of that name and that's familiar to you. When you see that person again, you'll remember his or her name because you've done this little exercise. This is especially beneficial to you if you are in a job or something similar where you must meet new people all the time.

You can also use music to help your memory. If you like a kind of music or you like to sing along to the lyrics of a favorite song, you probably don't struggle to remember those lyrics when you're singing them with the music. However, if you try to sing the lyrics to yourself without the music present, can you, do it? Try this; if there's a favorite song of yours that you like to sing along with all the time, try writing down the lyrics on your own, with no music present. After you finish, look at what you've done. Have parts of it like the chorus been easy to remember, while the verses may have been harder? Try again. Go from start to finish through the song as much as you can, writing down the lyrics as you go. Do this regularly, and you'll see how much music you remember. This is also a wonderful way to improve your memory.

The key to these brain exercises is that you have to find them fun, but challenging at the same time. If they're fun, you will look forward to doing them instead of avoiding them. And of course, since practice makes perfect, the more you do them, the more you'll see progress and improvement in your memory.

Basically, these types of exercises are a workout for your mind. You can always improve, no matter your age, and no matter how much trouble you may have recalling things at present. Remember that after about the age of 30, your mind can begin to lag a little bit cognitively. Don't wait until you notice detrimental changes to begin to do brain exercises. Start early so that you can retain mental sharpness even as you get older.

It can be challenging to improve your memory with these types of exercises, but it can also be fun. Try to do these activities daily, for at least 15 minutes. You'll be surprised at the improvement you see. And this is true no matter how old you are. If you "begin to lose memory," it can be short term in its duration, of course, but it can still cause frustration. So, give yourself the opportunity to gain a sharp memory that doesn't leave you in the dust when you need it most.

Helpful Tips for Improving Memory and Focus

Younger and younger people are complaining about memory problems. Many find it difficult to stay focused on anything for more than a few minutes at a time. If you are interested in improving your memory and focus, what can you do? Here are a few helpful tips that you can implement.

Creating the Right Circumstances for Remembering

Let's start with memory. Really the two-work hand in hand though. A key to memory is being focused. You need to pay attention to what it is that you want to remember, whether it be a name, a phone number, or a grocery list.

Repetition is another key to memory. Repeating something out loud, writing it down on a calendar or a to-do list, and even telling someone else about what you have to remember are all positive memory aids.

Associations and comparisons are also powerful memory tools. If you learn something new, the best way to remember it is to make a connection with something that you already knew. Compare or contrast your previous beliefs on the subject.

Finally, you can use certain memory aids such as a mind palace, a mnemonic device, or a means of organizing thoughts such as chronologically, alphabetically, or by subject.

Develop the Ability to Focus

Now let's talk focus. One of the biggest problems with focus today is that there is always something to distract us. The TV is on. Our cell phone is buzzing in our pocket. The tablet is chiming that a new message has arrived. Finding time for peace and quiet is vital for focus. A quiet room is best, but noise canceling headphones will do in a pinch. You can try some soothing music such as classical music (which is also good for memory and learning coincidentally).

Often, lack of sleep is a person's greatest obstacle to focus. Be sure to get a proper night's rest each night. This allows your mind the time it needs to clear out unnecessary stuff. With that done, your brain won't have so much crowding out your thoughts during the day.

Diet and exercise can also influence focus. While it is true that too much exercise can wear a person out and leave them too tired to think straight, a little cardio each day will keep blood flow to the brain at optimal levels. More oxygen means a brain that is running at its best capacity. Also, big meals can make you drowsy and affect focus. Try eating smaller meals more often. Too much sugar can also lead to a loss of focus, especially if your blood sugar spikes and then plummets, both of which are tough on the brain.

In the end, you may find that a combination of these factors is what you will need for improving memory and focus. Implement as many as possible, and see what works for you. Before long, your brain will be working like you've always wanted it

Free 25-minute meditation audio. Free Increasing Intelligence eBook, plus get the free 5-day intensive e-course on optimizing your intelligence and success in life special report from the author, click here.

Methods for Memory Improvement Based on Finding Your Best Learning Style

Our memory is so important since it helps us to keep those life events in our mind for the years to come. Of course, when you remember a memory from 15 years before but you forget the grocery list, it can be so irritating. There are many who want to find a way that they can improve upon their memory. Well, there are things you can do to help other than just dealing with frustration over things you forget.

It's important that we look at how things are learned before we get involved in methods for memory improvement. When you are involved in a new experience or you hear something new, the brain must take that information and decode it. It takes the information and interprets it in certain ways. When you are focusing on something and you learn something new, the brain takes the information and files it.

It is much like putting information into a file cabinet that you open. Once you want to remember that information again, the brain brings it out for you. It's just like walking back to the filing cabinet and retrieving the file you put in there before.

More than likely you can remember when your memory was great and you probably were used to that. When we don't work on keeping our brain in good shape and learning new ways that we can think, our memory skill may begin to slip a bit. Think of a dancer. While she may have spent time training for all her moves, when she stops training, she won't be able to get out there and start performing if she hasn't been practicing for many years. It's like that with the memory as well.

One way to improve memory is to constantly be aware of all that is going on around you. Many people only half listen when other people talk to them. It is easy to focus on another thing that you need to do instead of what they say. Make sure you start focusing on what is going on around you so you can store it and bring it back up in the future.

When you get additional information, work to associate it with something that you already know to make it easier to remember. There are a variety of different learning methods, so find the one that works out for you. There are some people that remember best when they have visual aids to help. Others learn best from hearing things. When you figure out your own learning style, you can work on it further to help improve your memory.

If you don't know something, find out more about it by researching it on your own. While it may seem difficult to learn, if you find a different way of learning it or a different explanation it may make more sense to you. Doing the research on something new helps you to acquire more knowledge, which will help you figure out which things you need to keep in your mind.

When you really want to ensure something is remembered, think about it and throw it around in your brain a few times. The more you repeat something in your mind, the better you'll learn it and be able to recall it in the future. Using visual aids and even word association can help with your memory too. Use the various memory aids available to help improve your memory

Healing with Meditation and Its Effective Use to Help People

Meditation is one of the most effective alternative therapies. In other words, it can be described as a mind-body medicine that has help several individuals throughout the world get relief from the symptoms of asthma, high blood pressure, insomnia, angina and stress. Besides, even the doctors believe of *healing with meditation* and its effectiveness recommending it to their patients.

Meditation is the safest and easiest means of balancing the mental, emotional and physical state of an individual. In fact, regardless of age, gender or medical condition, anybody can do it and reap its benefits. Though, it may sound like a new form of alternative therapy, it has its roots in ancient cultures and religions of the world. People have been practicing it throughout the ages all around the world.

Almost all the religious sects of the world practice meditation in one form or another. Besides, since ancient times, people have known about the healing by meditation. Even science has proved that medication works. Some of the known benefits of medication are calmness, blissful nature, peace of mind, overall good health, stress relief meditation, etc.

The Power of Healing with Meditation

Today, we can call meditation as a form of stress management which can help in creating constant positive energy to help our mind stay calm and battle the negative thoughts and outside elements that steal our peace. It helps a person to control his/her thoughts and emotions. In fact, an experienced meditation practitioner can have a higher level of control over such emotions, which helps him to turn negative energy into positive and better deal with it when faced with adversities.

In other words, it helps the individual to have a better control over his life since he can change the state of his mind whenever faced with challenges. Meditation is known to be beneficial in many ways. Today, stress is one of the most common issues we face, which plays a major role in being the cause of several ailments. However, meditation is the best treatment for reducing stress, and less stress means lesser problems.

Most of the people get overwhelmed by their immediate feelings and can't control their reactions, which further escalates the already bad situation into worse. However, with meditation one can easily manage anger & stress, and prevent such situations. The power to connect mind with the body and removing all the clutter from the mind helps in creating a medium for better spiritual atonement.

Most of the medical conditions can cause quite a pain and suffering. However, in some of the cases when the pain is mild, our mind can in fact amplify the pain and make it more excruciating. This can later act as a hindrance for the healing process and make it worse. As a matter of fact, studies have revealed that the healing with mediation sessions can help a person feel better by focusing more on the pleasant things rather than the pain. By doing so, the person can feel less pain or suffering and can reach a state where things become manageable.

One of the most noteworthy benefits of mediation is that it is quite effective in controlling the blood pressure. In fact, there's a type of meditation which is specifically meant for treating blood pressure issues.

Using meditation as a way of controlling the blood pressure also comes with an additional advantage and that is low dependence on drugs and strong pills.

Moreover, meditation even helps in developing a perpetual relaxation state, which later turns into routine practice whenever one feels uneasy or faces adverse situations. Bad or negative energies will always surround us; however, it is up to us to learn how to control it using positive energy.

Step by Step Guide to Begin Using Breathing Meditation to Relax the Mind, Focus

Commonly, the process of breathing meditation is designed to calm the mind and enhance the potential for inner peace. Many will opt to use breathing meditation to partially or totally reduce the levels of distractions that might be manifesting.

Meditation - The Easy Breathing Process

At the early stage of meditation, you will need to block any and all distractions which seek to undermine the ability to correctly meditate and allow the brain to think clearer and more coherently. Easy breathing meditation may make this more possible. We will need a calm place to meditate and the position you sit in must be comfortable. The traditional cross-legged position is preferred by many although you could employ any one of a number of other poses as well. You could even sit in a chair. The key point here is you need to keep your back unbent to keep the mind from getting sleepy or sluggish.

We will sit with our eyes partly shut and out attention will be turned inwards. We will breath naturally and through the nostrils and do so without any attempts to control our breath and take steps to develop a cognitive sense of our breathing as it enters and exists the nostrils. The aim of our meditation is to feel these sensations. Attention should be centered on it more than anything else when we meditate.

At first, our brain may be quite active and we might even feel that performing meditation makes our brain more active; yet, what is really happening is that we are using meditation to gain a clear insight into how active our brain has become. A great deal of temptation will arise nudging us to examine all the different thoughts that travel through our brain and we need to take the steps to resist their influence and stay focused on our breathing. If our brain starts to wander and our thoughts begin to meander, we need to return our attention on our breath and continue to meditate.

Repeat this as many times as possible until the mind concentrates on the proper task.

Those that take the time out to rehearse the process in a patient manner can lessen the impact of distracting thoughts effectively which may lead towards eventual inner peace. The mind will become more coherent in its thoughts and it will be free of much agitation and aggravation. Consider this similar to how an ocean will suffer from murkiness when water churns incessantly and the wind blows severely. To a degree, the endless flow of troubled thoughts can be quieted when we center on our breath and allow the mind to become clear and calm. It is advised to maintain this state of mind as much as possible.

While breathing meditation may only be a preliminary phase of meditation, it has a great many benefits associated with it. You might soon discover that taking part in the practice of meditation helps a person maintain a level of inner peace since the activities of the mind will be under greater personal control.

As soon as the troubling presence of disquieting thoughts diminishes and the brain becomes still, a greater sense of happiness and contentment will manifest from inside ourselves. This feeling of great contentment and well-being allows us to more effectively deal with those aspects of life we might not always find very enjoyable. A great deal of tension and stress we experience derives from our thoughts and many the issues we have to deal with such as physical health ailments will be increased by the stress we undergo. We will experience a calming, spacious feeling in the brain, and many problems we have to suffer through will diminish. Problematic and troubling situations will become a lot easier to address and we will begin to feel more positive as a result which will improve our relationships with others.

Practicing Mindfulness Meditation with Simple Techniques for Home and Work

Practicing Mindfulness

Mindfulness meditation can be done anywhere, but finding a quiet place makes it easier when you first begin. Sit comfortably. Begin focusing on each part of your body beginning with your feet. Tighten the muscle and hold it for a few seconds before moving on to your legs and upper body. Feel the tension lessening as you release. Work your way up to your hands and arms. When you have finished, focus on your breathing. One breathing technique that is helpful is to breath in for six seconds, hold the air in your lungs six seconds, exhale for six seconds, hold the breath out of your lungs for six seconds and repeat. The goal of these beginning exercises is to quiet the mind by putting all your focus on something else.

Next, find a word or phrase that is calming to you such as "inner peace". Repeat the word in your mind or say it aloud if you wish. Your mind might wonder, and that is alright. Gently bring your thoughts back to the phrase. Pay attention to how you feel when certain thoughts cross through. Are they uncomfortable? Do they help you in any way? If they are causing despair or anxiety then consider why for a moment, and then let them go. The point of mindfulness is to begin to control your thoughts and feelings instead of letting them control you.

The Most Effective Mindfulness Techniques for Busy Schedules

These Mindfulness techniques are simple, convenient, and effective, these can be used anywhere at any time to battle the daily stress we all encounter.

Deep Breathing

One of the best mindfulness techniques used in stress management is deep breathing. Something that can be done at work or home, it simply involves breathing from the stomach and making sure you inhale through your nose and exhale through your mouth. Not only will the physical act of deep breathing help to slow down your heart rate and keep the stress hormones in check, but it will also help clear the mind by letting you focus on the breathing itself. By closing your eyes and concentrating on the sound and rhythm of the breathing, you can calm down very quickly.

The Sound of Music

While music can soothe the savage beast, it can also be very therapeutic physically and emotionally. Whether it's classical music from Beethoven or the latest pop hit from the Billboard charts, music has been proven to be a great stress reliever. By focusing on the sounds and vibrations of each note and the feelings they generate within you, it's possible to clear out any negative thoughts you may be experiencing and replace them with positive ones.

House Cleaning

The notable thing about this technique is that you accomplish two things at the same time. Not only do you clear your mind and focus only on what's happening now, but you also get a clean house in the process. This is considered a great mindfulness technique because you can focus on so many distinct aspects. For example, when you are filling a box full of items to donate to charity, you can focus on clearing out the clutter in your own mind. If you're washing dishes, you can focus on how the warm, soapy water feels as you wash each dish, or let the vibrations from a vacuum cleaner soothe your mind.

Benefits of Mindfulness

Learning to control how you think and feel has many positive effects towards an increased ability to concentrate and focus on yourself instead of the negativity of others. By practicing mindfulness techniques daily, you'll quickly find yourself feeling less stressful and more positive about each day. Consider setting aside time each day for mindfulness meditation. Make the time for yourself one without judgment. The benefits of consistent mediation include decreased blood pressure, reduced anxiety and stress, and feelings of calmness. With practice, the reduced amount of time it takes to push negative thoughts away during mediation will decrease until you can quickly shut out thoughts that are distressing.

Advanced Meditation Techniques

It is a promising idea for regular practitioners of meditation, to give advanced meditation a try to get a better experience. Deeper meditation has greater benefits than just getting rid of stress. However, you can't perform these techniques without the correct guidance. These techniques give you more than just physical relaxation. They help in relaxing the subconscious mind too.

It is not easy for any beginner to perform advance techniques, as advanced meditation is quite complicated and long. It requires people who are having superior meditation abilities to be able to attain a unification with the universal energy and the powerful spiritual bliss, which begins to flow from them and spread onto the other people.

Meditation practices meant for beginners help you to clear your mind of thoughts. It also helps you to get rid of the stress and woes of your day to day life. As you move ahead towards the advanced meditation stages you will have to use your experience to resolve any stresses and issues in an active manner. The advanced techniques train you in setting aside the conscious mind and move ahead.

Deep meditation creates the route for the internal subconscious mind to get ahead and the brainwaves are restricted to less than the normal sleeping limits. This process is not at all easy and you should be prepared mentally to begin implementing these advanced techniques.

It is very important to be able to remain focused and prepared for a long session where you are not allowed to dose off.

If you wish to get better clarity on advanced meditation, you should relate your brain to an onion where all the layers are formed during your life, beginning from the time of birth.

Just like an onion, our brain too has various layers. The internal core of the onion is like our instinctual and primary segments of your brain and they make us aware of our thirst, sleep requirements, hunger, process of swallowing and blinking. These sections are also related to virtuous and pure.

This layer is followed by the childhood brain which stores the mastered behavior patterns and life experiences. Often this section is full of clutter and problems which does not let them view life in the proper aspects. In fact, these people do not even know about the true perspective of life.

This area makes us work very hard and you need to really struggle to focus on this area. Advance meditation stresses on this area effectively. You can compare the external layers of the onions to the adult brain. The outer skin can be compared to the conscious mind which is always cluttered with numerous stresses and thoughts. You need to tend to each layer carefully and the advanced meditation techniques are ideal for holistic healing.

After successfully moving through the basic levels you are ready to begin the practice of advanced meditation techniques. In a nutshell, if you wish to attain a higher level of consciousness then it is important to try advanced meditation.

Affiliate Marketing Online Business is Perfect Home Business for Injured and Disabled People

My personal experience of living disabled, a single parent for years and while working for now over the past 30 years since coming out of a coma after a serious accident has proven to me the value for individuals who are disabled in how much better it is to work from home in your own online business or as an affiliate marketer. I have tried several ways to earn income at home and recommend strongly the affiliate marketing sector of online businesses either part time or full time. Enjoy the article and blessings to you.

An accident, head injury and spinal cord injury in my early twenties changed my live drastically and fortunately I recovered enough to look at innovative ways of earning an income. Over the past twenty plus years, I've had technical training as part of rehabilitation that led to a successful career. However, the detrimental effects of the injuries worsened as I aged, leading to me being unable to work even at a desk or extended amounts of time. An 8-hr. day and 40 hour plus week just wore me out physically and even worsened the muscle weakness from the hemi-paresis, muscle weakness on one side that I had.

So now I was looking at earning income from home in several ways. I first tried selling on eBay but packing and shipping a high volume was not possible for me with my physical limitations. Then there was a serious communication issue when I tried several network marketing companies. The sometimes-slurred speech of mine ruined phone conversations and face to face meetings certainly did not show self-confidence or leadership skills. I also tried creating and selling digital products but the head injury certainly slowed me down and by the time I would create eBooks, websites, and launch the product, there were dozens of people selling a similar product or the ideas were outdated.

I found selling affiliate products was very easy for me, required no physical effort other than reading, a computer connection, 'one finger' typing and time. What I like best is that the computer did the communication. Sure, I had to set up the ad or webpage (and there is software for that even), but once I did the computer replicated my presentation flawlessly, thousands of times and my affiliate marketing online business was now paying me more than I earned from my past full-time job.

Basically, an affiliate marketing online business can be run from anywhere and I even started part time. You can of course earn a full-time income or even become a super affiliate earning a six-figure income. There is no inventory to stock in an affiliate marketing online business. Having a part of me disabled from an accident, I am excited about not having to pack and ship any products. You see the merchants that I represent or refer do all the work. They even collect the payments, processing credit cards worldwide so I have no payments to collect

Customer support is a big part of many businesses and their success. Some people must hire help or outsource this. Well not me in my affiliate marketing online business, the companies I refer do this work too. And best of all, many of these companies make payment immediately. Some wait 30 days when they have money back guarantees. But usually I get a PayPal payment right away or a transfer into my bank account either weekly or monthly. Some people still prefer checks delivered by snail mail. Well, they still do that too.

Having the right information and strategy is important to your success in affiliate marketing. If you set up your ads or website or ad or even articles as this one, your affiliate business will run itself. Sure, you may put in some time to build a site or write some ads but once they go live on the internet, you can go swimming, or as I do, just workout at the gym which I needed for ongoing rehabilitation. If you don't need either of these activities, then just watch the football game or spend time with friends as your affiliate income is deposited in your bank.

An important note is that the time spent setting these affiliate marketing websites, blogs or ads up does not have to be done at one time. Instead of two full 8 hr. workdays, a half hour or hour spread out over a couple weeks at a time is sufficient. For some disabled as I, this time benefit of an affiliate marketing online business is a real blessing... like gold.

By the way, you don't have to be disabled in any way to be have a successful affiliate business!

Learn Step by Step Free how to succeed online in an affiliate marketing online business. http://homebusinessit.com

At website, learn details of an affiliate marketing online business with articles, affiliate tools, video training and resources.

Successfully Golfing After a Stroke for Fun and Fitness

There are no denying stroke survivors have a lot to deal with as they go through the rehabilitation process and learn to live with physical limitations. Unfortunately, far too many people treat having a stroke as a sign they can no longer enjoy physical activities. For stroke survivors who love to play golf, those so-called physical limitations aren't as pronounced as one would imagine.

Playing Golf Again is a Real Possibility

Except in the worst of cases, the only thing that keeps most stroke survivors from getting back onto the golf course is the assumption they can't do it. That assumption is wrong in so many ways. Will their golf game be as proficient as it was before the stroke? Probably not, but everything in life changes after medical trauma. The reality is golf courses aren't going anywhere and any golfer who wants to golf belongs on the golf course. That includes stoke victims who love the game.

It only takes three things to make it happen. First, the person affected by the stroke must believe they can do it. Second, they need to accept certain limitations and learn to play within themselves. Finally, the stroke victim needs to minimize expectations and maximize the joy that comes from being out on a golf course instead of lying in a bed feeling disabled.

The Benefits of Golfing for Stroke Survivors

The benefits of being able to return to the golf course will touch almost every aspect of the stroke survivor's being. From a physical standpoint, they get the health benefits of fresh air and exercise. Doctors often encourage stroke victims to exercise their muscles and get the heart beating again. The walking and swinging of a club help to move all the right muscles and bring balance and coordination back.

As far as mental and emotional issues are concerned, there is nothing that revitalizes the spirit and soul more than overcoming impossible odds to achieve something important. If a golfer loves to golf, then learning to do it again under a separate set of circumstances is an accomplishment that should bring a profound sense of pride to a disabled golfer. In many cases, depression is a bigger threat to one's well-being than another stroke. By going out there on the golf course and proving they are still a player, the afflicted individual won't feel so afflicted anymore.

Finally, there is excellent value is participating in a social activity for a stroke survivor who has been hospitalized and/or confined to the home for a period. The chance to get out among friends and golfing buddies serves to make the person feel they are still a part of life here on this planet.

Exercises Designed to Make Golfing Easier for the Stroke Victim

While contemplating that first post-stroke round of golf, there are several exercises that can help reestablish stamina, balance and coordination. Walking is a must. Even cart riders will log distance during a round of golf. By getting out each day for a walk, it will improve endurance on the golf course. For balance and coordination, doctors recommend sitting on a stability ball but for those affected by stroke, a physical therapist should be close by unless one has progressed. By doing this exercise for just a few minutes every day, one's balance and ability to control their arms and legs will show marked improvement over time. A more sensible exercise at home would involve use of a chair. While the person affected by the stroke stands in a corner of a room, they hold on the back of the chair and practice moving hips forward and back and from side to side. This is also beneficial for strengthening the weakened side. If the survivor also has *foot drop* which many stroke victims experience, a brace recommended by the persons doctor for safety. It can help immensely as even if a cart is used, as the walking can tire out the weakened leg quickly at times.

Making Golf Easier for Stroke Survivors

The golfing world is well-aware that some stroke victims love the game of golf. With that in mind, there are plenty of custom equipment designers who are more than happy to help design golf equipment that compliments a golfer's disabilities. Another way golf is made easier for stroke victims is the process of making them feel normal. Disabled golfers are often reluctant to play golf with healthy people for fear of slowing the group down. First, golf is a game of courtesy and golfers tend to be very patient with those who might not be as skilled as the others in the group. That said, there are many golf courses that sponsor groups that have disabilities. By playing golf with other disabled golfers, the individual doesn't feel it necessary to perform, only to enjoy the outing.

Golf is a great sport and activity. If you or someone you know has suffered a stroke and would still love to hit the links, make it happen. With reasonable expectations, that first round of golf will feel like a rebirth of sorts, prompting the stroke victim to stop feeling like a victim and more as a winning survivor.

Watch free golf fitness and exercise videos online at the author's golf video website that target specific muscle groups used in your golf game, improving body motion or flexibility. These video tips, techniques, drills are from local and pro golf trainers, proven to improve aspects of your game and eliminating several bad golf playing habits. Visit http://golfworkoutsonline.com

Author Leon Edward at his website http://www.Hemiparesisliving.com presents articles. free resources, Checklists and tips from well-known professionals and authors in the field plus blogs on his own experiences with over 30 years living and working with hemiparesis. Persons and their families will benefit from the information on this site whether they have had a stroke, head injury as the author has, or other condition that caused partial or even full paralysis on one side of the body.

Additional References not previously mentioned

Deutsch. "Stroke." American Physical Therapy Association, 10 May 2011. Web. 21 Apr. 2015.
http://www.moveforwardpt.com/SymptomsConditions.

"Hemiparesis." *Stroke.org*. National Stroke Association, 16 July 2014. Web. 22 Apr. 2015.
http://stroke.org/we-can-help/survivors/stroke-recovery/post-stroke-conditions/physical/hemiparesis

O'Sullivan, Susan B, Schmitz, Thomas J. *Physical Rehabilitation.* 5th ed. Philadelphia: F.A. Davis, 2007, Print.

Rosamond et al. "AHA Statistical Update: Heart Disease and Stroke Statistics- 2007 Update." The American Heart Association. Web. 22 Apr. 2015.
http://circ.ahajournals.org/content/115/5/e69.full

Helpful Resources websites forums and blogs

- HELPFUL RESOURCES FORUMS SUPPORT GROUPS WEBSITES FACEBOOK GROUP TWITTER PAGES BLOGS OF INJURED, GUIDES AND BOOKS
    - Please visit http://hemiparesisliving.com/helpful-resources/

Resources are updated and added as recommended,

ABOUT THE AUTHOR

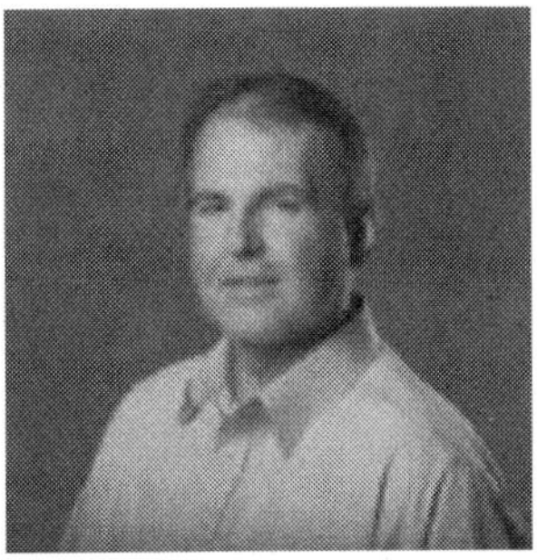

Description from SelfGrowth.com where his articles are published regularly on many categories of self-improvement and health.

Leon Edward, About

B.S. M. E., C.R.E, C.Q.A., C.Q.E.

Mind Brain Health Expert Author Leon Edward helps others keep their brain healthy, optimizing brain function at any age and maintain health aging of mind body and finances. He committed himself to optimizing the brain, mind power and healthy aging at conscious and subconscious levels after recovering from a serious neck and head injury from a gunshot at an early age. With an accredited Bachelors of Science in Mechanical Engineering from S.U.N.Y. followed by graduate study at RIT in Management and Applied Statistics, he went on to study cognitive thought processes and the power of the mind. After a successful 25-year career, he shares information on improving the mind freely as tips and the latest breakthroughs in mind power. He also provides health tips for similarly injured victims at his hemiparesis website.

Leon Edward helps people improve IQ, focus, memory, concentration, creativity, speed reading, public speaking, time management while reducing stress. Download his IQ Mind Brain Memory Self-Help library at his Brain Improvement website http://www.IQMindBrainLibrary.com

Leon Edward has published material on successfully living and working with Hemiparesis and Life after TBI or traumatic brain injury. His articles and featured guest articles can be read on recovery, rehabilitation and living injured at http://www.hemiparesisliving.com .

Leon Edward also helps others achieve personal and professional success, achievement of dreams and goals through mind control, creative visualization, universal laws, subconscious programming, hypnosis. Leon Edward helps people in Career Development, Finding Employment in a poor economy, Leadership, Goal Setting, Success, Motivation, Self-Improvement, Happiness, Memory Improvement, Stress Reduction and more at his Personal Development Training and Living Successfully website LeonEdward.com . Stay current with the latest creativity news, workshops and training at his Creativity and Innovation website, http://www.creativityoverdrive.com

Made in the USA
Las Vegas, NV
13 February 2021

17790443R00090